ATI TEAS: Workbook Containing 6 Full-Length Practice Tests

Library of Congress Cataloging-in-Publication Data
Smart Edition Media.

ATI TEAS: Workbook Containing 6 Full-Length Practice Tests.
ISBN: 978-1-949147-65-0

1. ATI TEAS.
2. Study Guides.
3. TEAS
4. Nursing
5. Careers

Disclaimer:

The opinions expressed in this publication are the sole works of Smart Edition Media and were created independently from any National Evaluation Systems or other testing affiliates. Between the time of publication and printing, specific standards as well as testing formats and website information may change that are not included in part or in whole within this product. Smart Edition Media develops sample test questions, and they reflect similar content as on real tests; however, they are not former tests. Smart Edition Media assembles content that aligns with exam standards but makes no claims nor guarantees candidates a passing score.

Printed in the United States of America

ATI TEAS: Workbook Containing 6 Full-Length Practice Tests/Smart Edition Media.

ISBN: Print: 978-1-949147-65-0
     Ebook: 978-1-949147-66-7

Print and digital composition by Book Genesis, Inc.

HOW TO ACCESS THE ONLINE RESOURCES

To access your online resources, follow these instructions:

1. Go to www.smarteditionmedia.com.
2. Select Sign In in the website navigation at the top of the page.
3. Select your book.
4. Follow the instructions on the login page for locating the password in your book (the password is case sensitive, so be sure to include any capital letters at the beginning of the password).

 Practice tests   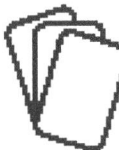 Flashcards    Videos

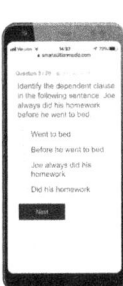

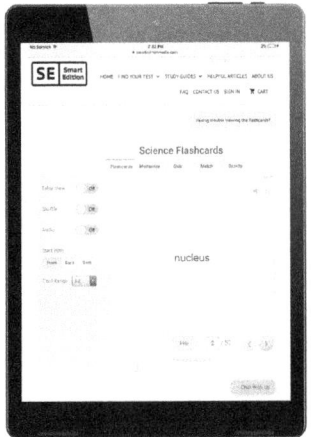

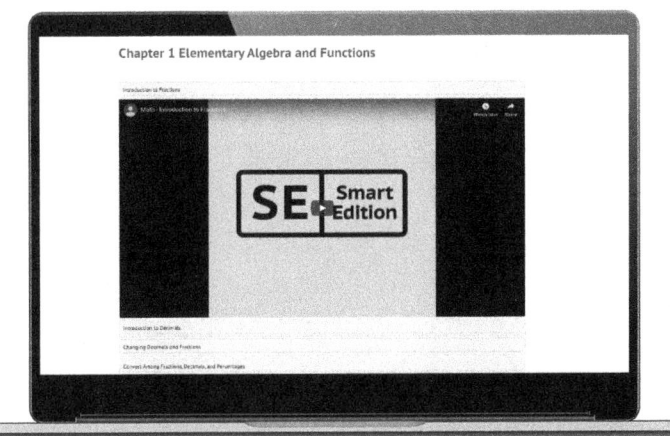

TABLE OF CONTENTS

INTRODUCTION

TEAS OVERVIEW

The Test of Essential Academic Skills (TEAS) is a standardized exam that is published by the Assessment Technologies Institute (ATI) Nursing Education. It is used as part of an overall assessment of qualifications for individuals when applying to a nursing school or an allied health school. Professionals already working in the health science industry may also take this exam while embarking on the path to advanced certification. The exam is administered weekly at PSI testing centers, as well as at nursing and allied health schools throughout the United States and Canada.

ABOUT THIS BOOK

This book provides you with an accurate and complete representation of the Test of Essential Academic Skills (TEAS) standardized exam and includes all four sections found on the exam: Reading, Mathematics, Science, and English Language and Usage.

The six full-length practice tests in the book are based on the TEAS and contain questions similar to those you can expect to encounter on the official test. A detailed answer key follows each practice test. These answer keys provide explanations designed to help you completely understand the test material.

ONLINE SAMPLE TESTS

The purchase of this book grants you access to digital versions of the six tests found in this book. This enables you the ultimate flexibility in creating a study plan that works with your lifestyle. Whether at home or on-the-go, you have full access to the materials you need to succeed in passing the test!

You can locate these exams on the Smart Edition Media website.

Go to the URL: https://smarteditionmedia.com/pages/teasworkbook-online-resources and follow the password/login instructions.

HOW TO USE THIS BOOK

Congratulations on taking the first steps to achieving your career goals! Thank you for allowing Smart Edition Media to accompany you on your journey to success.

Taking practice tests is a great way to familiarize yourself with the test format, question structure, and content of an exam. Each of the tests in this workbook identifies the amount of time allowed for each section of the actual exam and includes questions similar to those you are likely to see on the actual exam. By using a methodical approach to taking practice tests, you can significantly improve your accuracy and comfortability with this exam.

This workbook contains 6 full-length practice tests. As an added resource, we have made these same tests available to you electronically on our website. Whether you prefer to practice online or with paper and pencil, we've got you covered! The online test will provide you with a diagnostic report of your score that highlights areas of strength and weakness. In fact, it is worth entering your answers into the online test – even if you take it on paper – simply to get this report. To do so, just go to the online resources site, enter the answers you wrote in your workbook as you click through the test. The questions are static and will appear in exactly the same order online and in print – though you might want to spot check as you enter your answers just to be sure you have not missed a question.

HOW THIS BOOK IS ORGANIZED

STEP ONE: DETERMINE YOUR BASELINE SCORE.

We suggest taking one test first as a diagnostic tool to find your baseline score. Log on to https://smarteditionmedia.com/pages/teasworkbook-online-resources and follow the password/login instructions. Try to replicate actual test-taking conditions by working in a quiet location and adhering to the time limits of each section. Once completed, you will receive a diagnostic report that will help you to determine areas of strength and weakness.

STEP TWO: PRACTICE ENGAGED TEST-TAKING SKILLS.

For your second and third practice test, simulate the same quiet environment, but allow yourself more time to take each section.

- Make margin notes of questions that you find challenging: circle unfamiliar words, use question marks or asterisk to note concepts that you want to review, and write reminders to yourself as you go through the test.
- Keep in mind the results of your diagnostic test as you work. If you need more time on a particular section, take it! If it helps you to look up words in a dictionary or refer to facts in a textbook or other reference book, by all means, do so! You can find helpful study

tools, such as flashcards and subject-specific information sheets at the online resources page of the Smart Edition Media website listed above.

- Check your answers against the Answer Key and read through the Answer Explanations for any question that you answered incorrectly, referring back to your reference materials for further clarification, if necessary.

In these practice test scenarios, you should focus on completing as much as you can based on what you know and work through skills that might still be challenging by researching unfamiliar content as you go.

STEP THREE: SIMULATE THE ACTUAL TESTING ENVIRONMENT.

Once you have taken a few practice tests and worked through your targeted areas of difficulty, it is time to simulate the actual testing environment.

- Schedule time with yourself to take the test as if it were the actual test day. Circle the date on your calendar and get a good night's rest the night before.
- Set aside a quiet place to take the test, clearing away all reference materials and notes. Eat a well-balanced meal or healthy snack before sitting down to take the test, just like you would the morning of the exam.
- Select one of the remaining full-length practice tests, in this workbook or online, and adhere to the time limits posted for each section as you take the test. Check your answers against the Answer Key and read through the Answer Explanations for any question that you answered incorrectly, referring back to your reference materials for further clarification, if necessary.
- Evaluate the results of your tests, from the first to the last one that you have taken. Acknowledge the improvements that you have made throughout this process, and note any trouble spots that remain. Use this information to target your remaining study time before the exam.
- By the time you have worked through this process, the date of your actual exam is most likely drawing near. If you have followed this outline, you will have at least two full-length practice test remaining. Use these tests, either in sections or as a whole, as additional practice in the days preceding the actual test.
- Also note that the results of this process: the margin notes that you've taken, the questions and your answers, and the answer explanations, can be used as a personalized study guide to keep the core skills sharp. Flip through your work the day before the exam to refresh your memory. You have put diligent, focused effort into preparing for this exam. Congratulations on all your hard work!

** This TEAS Workbook contains 6 full-length practice tests (in print and online) and can be used alone or in conjunction with the TEAS Full Study Guide.

STUDY STRATEGIES AND TIPS

MAKE STUDY SESSIONS A PRIORITY.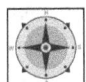

- Use a calendar to schedule your study sessions. Set aside a dedicated amount of time each day/week for studying. While it may seem difficult to manage, given your other responsibilities, remember that in order to reach your goals, it is crucial to dedicate the time now to prepare for this test. A satisfactory score on your exam is the key to unlocking a multitude of opportunities for your future success.
- Do you work? Have children? Other obligations? Be sure to take these into account when creating your schedule. Work around them to ensure that your scheduled study sessions can be free of distractions.

TIPS FOR FINDING TIME TO STUDY.
- Wake up 1-2 hours before your family for some quiet time
- Study 1-2 hours before bedtime and after everything has quieted down
- Utilize weekends for longer study periods
- Hire a babysitter to watch children

TAKE PRACTICE TESTS

- Smart Edition Media offers practice tests, both online and in print. Take as many as you can to help be prepared. This will eliminate any surprises you may encounter during the exam.

KNOW YOUR LEARNING STYLE

- Identify your strengths and weaknesses as a student. All students are different and everyone has a different learning style. Do not compare yourself to others.
- Howard Gardner, a developmental psychologist at Harvard University, has studied the ways in which people learn new information. He has identified seven distinct intelligences. According to his theory:

  "we are all able to know the world through language, logical-mathematical analysis, spatial representation, musical thinking, the use of the body to solve problems or to make things, an understanding of other individuals, and an understanding of ourselves. Where individuals differ is in the strength of these intelligences - the so-called profile of intelligences -and in the ways in which such intelligences are invoked and combined to carry out different tasks, solve diverse problems, and progress in various domains."

- Knowing your learning style can help you to tailor your studying efforts to suit your natural strengths.
- What ways help you learn best? Videos? Reading textbooks? Find the best way for you to study and learn/review the material

WHAT IS YOUR LEARNING STYLE?

- **Visual-Spatial** – Do you like to draw, do jigsaw puzzles, read maps, daydream? Creating drawings, graphic organizers, or watching videos might be useful for you.
- **Bodily-kinesthetic** – Do you like movement, making things, physical activity? Do you communicate well through body language, or like to be taught through physical activity? Hands-on learning, acting out, role playing are tools you might try.
- **Musical** – Do you show sensitivity to rhythm and sound? If you love music, and are also sensitive to sounds in your environments, it might be beneficial to study with music in the background. You can turn lessons into lyricsor speak rhythmically to aid in content retention.
- **Interpersonal** – Do you have many friends, empathy for others, street smarts, and interact well with others? You might learn best in a group setting. Form a study group with other students who are preparing for the same exam. Technology makes it easy to connect, if you are unable to meet in person, teleconferencing or video chats are useful tools to aid interpersonal learners in connecting with others.
- **Intrapersonal** – Do you prefer to work alone rather than in a group? Are you in tune with your inner feelings, follow your intuition and possess a strong will, confidence and opinions? Independent study and introspection will be ideal for you. Reading books, using creative materials, keeping a diary of your progress will be helpful. Intrapersonal learners are the most independent of the learners.
- **Linguistic** – Do you use words effectively, have highly developed auditory skills and often think in words? Do you like reading, playing word games, making up poetry or stories? Learning tools such as computers, games, multimedia will be beneficial to your studies.
- **Logical-Mathematical** – Do you think conceptually, abstractly, and are able to see and explore patterns and relationships? Try exploring subject matter through logic games, experiments and puzzles.

CREATE THE OPTIMAL STUDY ENVIRONMENT

- Some people enjoy listening to soft background music when they study. (Instrumental music is a good choice.) Others need to have a silent space in order to concentrate. Which do you prefer? Either way, it is best to create an environment that is free of distractions for your study sessions.
- Have study guide – Will travel! Leave your house: Daily routines and chores can be distractions. Check out your local library, a coffee shop, or other quiet space to remove yourself from distractions and daunting household tasks will compete for your attention.
- Create a Technology Free Zone. Silence the ringer on your cell phone and place it out of reach to prevent surfing the Web, social media interactions, and email/texting exchanges. Turn off the television, radio, or other devices while you study.
- Are you comfy? Find a comfortable, but not *too* comfortable, place to study. Sit at a desk or table in a straight, upright chair. Avoid sitting on the couch, a bed, or in front of the TV. Wear clothing that is not binding and restricting.
- Keep your area organized. Have all the materials you need available and ready: Smart Edition study guide, computer, notebook, pen, calculator, and pencil/eraser. Use a desk lamp or overhead light that provides ample lighting to prevent eye-strain and fatigue.

HEALTHY BODY, HEALTHY MIND

- Consider these words of wisdom from Buddha, "To keep the body in good health is a duty – otherwise we shall not be able to keep our mind strong and clear."

> **KEYS TO CREATING A HEALTHY BODY AND MIND:**
> - Drink water – Stay hydrated! Limit drinks with excessive sugar or caffeine.
> - Eat natural foods – Make smart food choices and avoid greasy, fatty, sugary foods.
> - Think positively – You can do this! Do not doubt yourself, and trust in the process.
> - Exercise daily – If you have a workout routine, stick to it! If you are more sedentary, now is a great time to begin! Try yoga or a low-impact sport. Simply walking at a brisk pace will help to get your heart rate going.
> - Sleep well – Getting a good night's sleep is important, but too few of us actually make it a priority. Aim to get eight hours of uninterrupted sleep in order to maximize your mental focus, memory, learning, and physical wellbeing.

FINAL THOUGHTS

- Remember to relax and take breaks during study sessions.
- Review the testing material. Go over topics you already know for a refresher.
- Focus more time on less familiar subjects.

EXAM PREPARATION

In addition to studying for your upcoming exam, it is important to keep in mind that you need to prepare your mind and body as well. When preparing to take an exam as a whole, not just studying, taking practice exams, and reviewing math rules, it is critical to prepare your body in order to be mentally and physically ready. Often, your success rate will be much higher when you are *fully* ready.

Here are some tips to keep in mind when preparing for your exam:

SEVERAL WEEKS/DAYS BEFORE THE EXAM

- Get a full night of sleep, approximately 8 hours
- Turn off electronics before bed
- Exercise regularly
- Eat a healthy balanced diet, include fruits and vegetable
- Drink water

THE NIGHT BEFORE

- Eat a good dinner
- Pack materials/bag, healthy snacks, and water

- Gather materials needed for test: your ID and receipt of test. You do not want to be scrambling the morning of the exam. If you are unsure of what to bring with you, check with your testing center or test administrator.
- Map the location of test center, identify how you will be getting there (driving, public transportation, uber, etc.), when you need to leave, and parking options.
- Lay your clothes out. Wear comfortable clothes and shoes, do not wear items that are too hot/cold
- Allow minimum of ~8 hours of sleep
- Avoid coffee and alcohol
- Do not take any medications or drugs to help you sleep
- Set alarm

THE DAY OF THE EXAM

- Wake up early, allow ample time to do all the things you need to do and for travel
- Eat a healthy, well-rounded breakfast
- Drink water
- Leave early and arrive early, leave time for any traffic or any other unforeseeable circumstances
- Arrive early and check in for exam. This will give you enough time to relax, take off coat, and become comfortable with your surroundings.

Take a deep breath, get ready, go! You got this!

TEAS Practice Exam 1

Section I. Reading

You have 64 minutes to complete 53 questions.

Please read the text below and answer questions 1-5.

Most people have had the pleasure of tasting a delicious chocolate chip cookie at some point in their lives. But what most folks do not know is that chocolate chip cookies were invented by accident. Ruth Graves Wakefield, owner of the popular Toll House Inn in Whitman, Massachusetts, prepared all the food for her guests. People came from all over to stay at the Toll House Inn and eat her famous Chocolate Butter Drop Do cookies. These chocolate cookies were such a hit that Ruth found herself baking them on a daily basis. One day, when she was preparing the recipe, she realized she had run out of baker's chocolate. She decided to break up a block of Nestle semi-sweet chocolate instead, expecting them to melt and disperse through the cookie dough. To her surprise, when she took the cookies out of the oven, the chocolate morsels retained their shape as "chips" in the cookie, thereby making them the first batch of chocolate chip cookies every baked. Ruth's chocolate chip cookies were so popular that they ended up permanently replacing her Chocolate Butter Drop Do cookies. Thanks to this happy accident, people all over the world get to enjoy one of the best desserts ever invented!

1. **Which sentence is the topic sentence?**

   A. Most people have had the pleasure of tasting a delicious chocolate chip cookie at some point in their lives.

   B. But what most folks do not know is that chocolate chip cookies were invented by accident.

   C. She decided to break up a block of Nestle semi-sweet chocolate instead, expecting them to melt and disperse through the cookie dough.

   D. Ruth's chocolate chip cookies were so popular that they ended up permanently replacing her Chocolate Butter Drop Do cookies.

2. **In the paragraph, the chocolate chip cookie is:**

   A. the topic.

   B. the main idea.

   C. a supporting detail.

   D. the topic sentence.

3. **Which sentence summarizes the main idea of the paragraph?**

   A. Chocolate chip cookies are more popular than Chocolate Butter Drop Do cookies.

   B. Ruth Graves Wakefield became famous for her chocolate chip cookie recipe.

   C. One of the most classic and popular desserts came about unexpectedly.

   D. It takes a whole lot of work to create something long-lasting.

4. **Which of the following sentences from the paragraph is a supporting detail of the topic sentence?**

   A. Ruth Graves Wakefield, owner of the popular Toll House Inn in Whitman, Massachusetts, prepared all the food for her guests on a daily basis.

   B. People came from all over to stay at the Toll House Inn and eat her famous Chocolate Butter Drop Do cookies.

   C. These chocolate cookies were such a hit that Ruth found herself baking them on a daily basis.

   D. She decided to break up a block of Nestle semi-sweet chocolate instead, expecting them to melt and disperse through the cookie dough.

5. **Which sentence would *best* function as a supporting detail in this paragraph?**

   A. The Nestle Company now owns the rights to Ruth Graves Wakefield's chocolate chip cookie recipe.

   B. Ruth Graves Wakefield tasted the cookies with the chocolate morsels in them and realized immediately how delicious they were.

   C. Today people buy pre-packaged chocolate chips instead of breaking off pieces of chocolate from a Nestle bar.

   D. Ruth Graves Wakefield sold her recipe in exchange for a lifetime of free chocolate.

Read the text below and answer question 6.

Before I came to America, I couldn't have known how difficult it would be. I knew I would miss my mother and my friends and my language, but I didn't know I would have to scrabble so desperately for so long to earn my place. Even when I had managed to make a living, I overworked myself with an animal terror. When I left home, I thought I was leaving poverty behind, but eventually I came to understand that I had escaped physical poverty by stepping into a poverty of the soul.

6. **Which sequence accurately describes what happened first, second, and third in the passage?**

   A. Arriving in America, overworking, escaping physical poverty

   B. Coming to America, escaping physical poverty, stepping into a poverty of the soul

   C. Knowing how difficult America would be, leaving home, stepping into a poverty of the soul

   D. Expecting to miss friends, knowing how difficult America would be, arriving in America

Read the following text and its summary and answer questions 7-8.

Text: In the late 1800s, life was terrible for some children. The Industrial Revolution was in full effect and factories sprang up in urban areas all over the country. Many innocent children left the comforts of home for the big cities to make money for their families. Children as young as 6 were forced to work long hours with dangerous equipment for little pay. A lot of children grew ill or even died on the job. Factory owners justified this abominable treatment by claiming they fed, clothed, and provided shelter for these children.

Summary: The author argues that children led awful lives during the Industrial Revolution due to long work hours, dangerous equipment, and little pay. Factory owners justified this treatment even though children were becoming ill or dying.

7. **Is this summary effective? Why or why not?**

   A. The summary is effective because it captures the emotional component of the text.

   B. The summary is effective because it restates the key points in a new way.

   C. The summary is ineffective because it makes its own claims and judgments.

   D. The summary is ineffective because it is structurally the same as the original.

8. **If the first line of the summary were replaced, which of the following lines would make the summary ineffective?**

   A. The author claims that in the late 1800s, life was terrible for some children.

   B. The author states that during the Industrial Revolution, children faced many hardships.

   C. The author claims that life was difficult for children during the Industrial Revolution.

   D. The author states that children who worked during the Industrial Revolution had it tough.

9. **Which of the following would make a summary ineffective?**

   A. One that is objective

   B. One that uses new words

   C. One full of the main ideas

   D. One that is structurally plagiarized

Read the following draft paragraph and answer questions 10-12.

(1) After you set up your drain pan, it's time to remove the drain plug. (2) Use your wrench to loosen the plug. (3) It helps to work slowly. (4) If possible, keep your hands and arms away from the stream. (5) This gets messy, so put on your gloves.

10. **Which change to the paragraph would make its organization more sequential?**

   A. Delete sentence 2.

   B. Move sentence 5 earlier.

   C. Switch sentences 2 and 3.

   D. Combine sentences 2 and 3.

11. **Which sentence combines the ideas from sentences 2 and 3 without changing the meaning?**

    A. Using your wrench, slowly loosen the plug.

    B. Using your wrench, the plug is slowly loosened.

    C. It helps to work slowly to loosen the plug after you use your wrench.

    D. It helps to work slowly to loosen the plug before you use your wrench.

12. **The writer is considering adding the following sentence to the paragraph.**

    The oil comes out fast, and if the car has been running recently, it can be hot.

    Where would it make the most sense to place this sentence?

    A. Before sentence 1

    B. After sentence 2

    C. After sentence 4

    D. After sentence 5

13. **What is revision?**

    A. Creating a mind map to organize ideas

    B. Correcting misspellings and grammatical errors

    C. Forming a question to guide the research process

    D. Strengthening the content and organization in writing

Read the following draft paragraph and answer questions 14-16.

DuMont High School should delay its start time so students can stay alert while they learn. (1) I read about a study that showed that teenagers need 8-9 hours of sleep per night to function optimally. (2) There was another study saying teenagers' bodies naturally stay up later at night and wake later in the morning than adults' bodies. (3) Therefore, the science proves that our current start time of 7:15 a.m. is damaging to students. (4) The school board is obviously trying to inflict cruel and unusual punishment on us. (5)

14. **How could the writer of the paragraph make the evidence presented in Sentence 2 and Sentence 3 more trustworthy?**

    A. By using a clear transition phrase

    B. By deleting the word *I* from the text

    C. By naming the study and its authors

    D. By explaining the meaning of *optimally*

15. **The point in Sentence 4 needs revision because:**

    A. many teenagers enjoy getting up early.

    B. the transition *therefore* is not effective.

    C. the start time mentioned is not accurate.

    D. the evidence does not clearly support it.

16. The emotional appeal in Sentence 5 is manipulative because it:

    A. uses a cliché phrase, "cruel and unusual punishment."

    B. attacks people who disagree with the author's argument.

    C. employs understatement to distract from an opposing point.

    D. exaggerates the consequences of refusing to accept the proposal.

17. **Read the sentences below.**

    Carla performed in the Boston Ballet Corps as a principal dancer in her twenties. She became a Broadway choreographer thereafter.

    Which word functions as a transition?

    A. twenties   C. became

    B. she   D. thereafter

18. **Read the sentences below.**

    Dogs are typically friendly, loyal animals that love people. <u>However,</u> some people train their dogs to be vicious fighters, so you should always ask pet owners if it's safe to approach their dog.

    What is the function of the <u>underlined</u> transition word in sentence two?

    A. To express a contrast

    B. To provide an example

    C. To add emphasis to a point

    D. To indicate time or sequence

Read the passage and answer questions 19-22.

Dear Mr. O'Hara,

I am writing to let you know how much of a positive impact you have made on our daughter. Before being in your algebra class, Violet was math phobic. She would shut down when new concepts would not come to her easily. As a result, she did not pass many tests. Despite this past struggle, she has blossomed in your class! Your patience and dedication have made all the difference in the world. Above all, your one-on-one sessions with her have truly helped her in ways you cannot imagine. She is a more confident and capable math student, thanks to you. We cannot thank you enough.

Fondly,

Bridgette Foster

19. **Which adjective best describes the tone of this passage?**

    A. Arrogant   C. Friendly

    B. Hopeless   D. Appreciative

20. **Which phrase from the passage has an openly appreciative and warm tone?**

    A. I am writing to let you now

    B. you have made on our daughter

    C. made all the difference

    D. We cannot thank you enough

21. **What mood would this passage most likely evoke in the math teacher, Mr. O'Hara?**

    A. Calm

    B. Grateful

    C. Sympathetic

    D. Embarrassed

22. **Which transition word or phrase from the passage adds emphasis to the writer's point?**

    A. Being

    B. As a result

    C. Despite

    D. Above all

23. **An author's purpose is the:**

    A. opinion the author has on a topic.

    B. reason an author writes something.

    C. strategies the author uses to entertain.

    D. details the author uses to explain a process.

Read the following text and answer questions 24-28.

Wizard WiFi is a digital application that allows you to manage your home WiFi network and connected devices. Wizard WiFi is easy to install and set up! Once installed Wizard WiFi enables you to find your WiFi password, know who is online, troubleshoot issues and manage family members' online experiences. You will be a tech-savvy genius in no time!

Concerned about creating healthy tech-usage habits? Wizard WiFi allows you to create individualized WiFi usage limits and alert family members when they are nearing their daily quota, set a "Bedtime Mode" to create an optimal "tech-free" nighttime environment, and ensure age-appropriate, safe Web surfing with features like Pause and Parental Controls. It is the best technology management system on the market! If you are a Wizard Internet subscriber with a SuperWiz Gateway, you can access the Wizard WiFi experience at no additional cost through a mobile app, website or an app on the SuperWiz TV Box. New Wizard Internet subscribers

can access Wizard WiFi once their SuperWiz Gateway is activated. Existing subscribers with eligible SuperWiz Gateways can log into the Wizard WiFi portal immediately.

Top-level high-tech executives, like Pear Technology CEO Rusty Bartlett, rely on Wizard WiFi to manage the safety and security of their home WiFi network systems. Shouldn't you do the same?

24. **The purpose of this passage is to:**

    A. decide.

    B. inform.

    C. persuade.

    D. entertain.

25. **With which statement would the author of this passage most likely agree?**

    A. People who have home WiFi networks use excessive technology and do not value spending quality time with family members.

    B. Parents who do not buy WiFi monitoring devices are unable to have confidence in the security of their household network.

    C. The best way to achieve a healthy tech environment is to create family rules for technology usage and avoid monitoring apps.

    D. Consumers want help managing their home technology systems to create healthy habits and ensure a secure and safe online environment for family members.

26. **Which detail from the passage, if true, is factual?**

    A. Wizard WiFi transforms the user into a tech-savvy genius.

    B. Wizard WiFi is the best technology-management system on the market.

    C. Wizard WiFi products contain functions that set and track individual users' technology usage.

    D. Wizard WiFi users will improve the way their family spends their technology-free quality time.

27. **The author of the passage includes details about Wizard WiFi's ease of use in order to appeal to the reader's:**

    A. trust.   C. feelings.

    B. reason.   D. knowledge.

28. **The author most likely includes the detail about a famous high-tech executive CEO in order to make readers:**

    A. understand that Wizard WiFi is factually the best on the market.

    B. take a weak position when they attempt to argue against the point.

    C. trust that Information Technology professionals have really studied Wizard WiFi and proven it worthy.

    D. feel an association between Wizard WiFi products and a person they admire.

29. **Which of the following is not a formatting feature?**

    A. Italics   C. Boldfacing

    B. Charts   D. Underlining

30. **An argument may be composed of:**

    A. facts only.

    B. opinions only.

    C. both facts and opinions.

    D. neither facts nor opinions.

31. **Which sentence does *not* display gender bias?**

    A. Ask a police officer for directions, and she will help you arrive at your destination safely.

    B. Ask a police officer for directions, and the police officer will help you arrive at your destination safely.

    C. Ask a police officer for directions, and they will help you arrive at your destination safely.

    D. Ask a police officer for directions, and he will help you arrive at your destination safely.

32. **Which of the following sources should be treated with skepticism even though it is primary?**

    A. The field notes of a scientist studying primate behavior in the wild

    B. A diary of a child who operated a loom in the Lowell Mills

    C. An interview with a ninety-two-year-old Holocaust survivor

    D. An article from the turn of the 19th century about the best farming practices

Study the following label and answer questions 33-36.

Nutrition Facts

Serving Size 20 crackers (38g)
Servings Per Container 5

Amount Per Serving

Calories 150   Calories from Fat 45

	% Daily Value*
Total Fat 9g	**12%**
Saturated Fat 4g	**20%**
Trans Fat 0g	
Cholesterol 0mg	**0%**
Sodium 160mg	**7%**
Total Carbohydrate 16g	**6%**
Dietary Fiber Less than 1g	**2%**
Sugars Less than 1g	**0%**
Protein 1g	
Vitamin D	0%
Calcium	5%
Iron	20%
Potassium	8%

* Percent Daily Values are based on a 2,000 calorie diet. Your Daily Values may be higher or lower depending on your calorie needs:

	Calories:	2,000	2,500
Total Fat	Less than	65g	80g
Saturated Fat	Less than	20g	25g
Cholesterol	Less than	300mg	300mg
Sodium	Less than	2,400mg	2,400mg
Total Carbohydrate		300g	375g
Dietary Fiber		25g	30g

33. **How many calories are in one serving of this product?**

   A. 5   C. 150

   B. 20   D. 3,750

34. **Germain ate 60 crackers out of this box. How many servings did he consume?**

   A. 1   C. 5

   B. 3   D. 10

35. **The product in this package is considered high in:**

   A. sodium.   C. cholesterol.

   B. trans fat.   D. saturated fat.

36. **Fatima is attempting to confine her diet to products low in sodium. How much of this product should she eat?**

   A. None; the product is not low in sodium.

   B. One serving; the amount of sodium is reasonable.

   C. The whole package; the contents are appropriate for a low-sodium diet.

   D. Less than three servings; she needs to keep her sodium intake below 20%.

37. **The product in this package is a good source of:**

   A. iron.   C. calcium.

   B. fiber.   D. vitamin D.

Read the following paragraphs and answer questions 38-41.

The idea of getting rid of homework at the elementary school level is debatable, but giving young children a well-needed break after school is undoubtedly beneficial. A study of elementary-age children and homework showed that daily homework causes high rates of anxiety and depression in young people. In contrast, schools that have gotten rid of the homework requirement have reported a drop in depression and anxiety among students.

According to a nationwide analysis of standardized testing scores, schools that have gotten rid of homework have seen benefits. Test scores have gone up incrementally from year to year. On the contrary, schools that mandate daily homework have seen stagnant test scores. Therefore, it is safe to say that homework does nothing to enhance student learning at all.

38. **Which statement expresses an opinion?**

   A. The idea of getting rid of homework at the elementary school level is debatable, but giving young children a well-needed break after school is undoubtedly beneficial.

   B. A study of elementary-age children and homework showed that daily homework causes high rates of anxiety and depression in young people.

   C. In contrast, schools that have gotten rid of the homework requirement have reported a drop in depression and anxiety among students.

   D. According to a nationwide analysis of standardized testing scores, schools that have gotten rid of homework have seen benefits.

39. **Consider the following sentence from the passage:**

   On the contrary, schools that mandate daily homework have seen stagnant test scores.

   Is this statement a fact or an opinion? Why?

   A. An opinion because it focuses on the beliefs of the schools involved

   B. An opinion because it expresses how the author feels about standardized test scores

   C. A fact because it shares test score results, which are something that can be verified

   D. A fact because it relies on the schools' projected test score results

40. **What is the primary argument of the passage?**

   A. Schools need to change the type of homework they give to elementary school students.

   B. There are no clear benefits from giving elementary-aged students daily homework.

   C. A school's standardized test scores are a good measure of how the school is performing overall.

   D. Schools with stagnant test scores would benefit from giving students more homework.

41. **Which sentence in the passage displays faulty reasoning?**

   A. According to a nationwide analysis of standardized testing scores, schools that have gotten rid of homework have seen benefits.

   B. Test scores have gone up incrementally from year to year.

   C. On the contrary, schools that mandate daily homework have seen stagnant test scores.

   D. Therefore, it is safe to say that homework does nothing to enhance student learning at all.

Study the infographic below and answer questions 42-44.

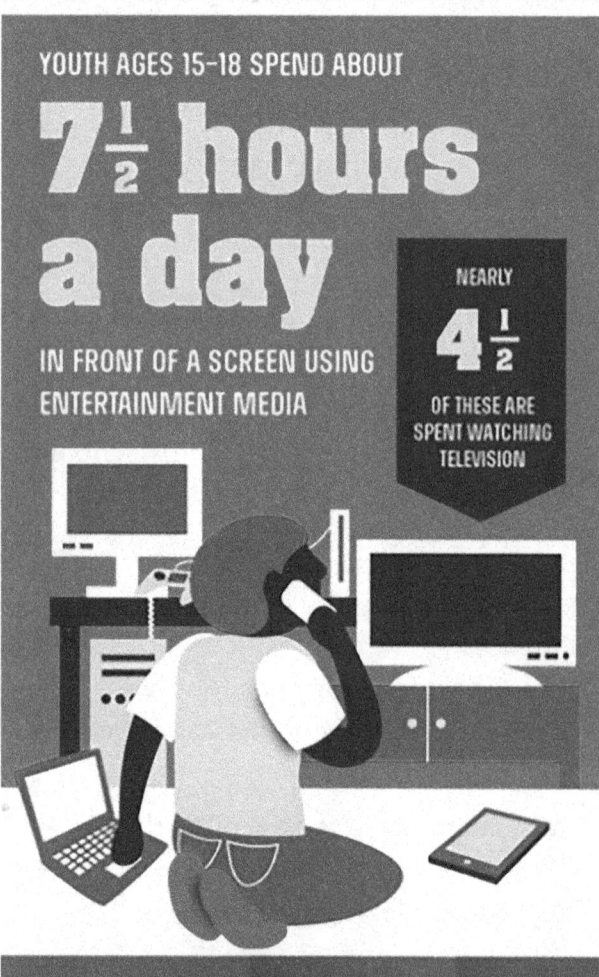

SCREEN TIME VS LEAN TIME

Do you know how much entertainment screen time kids get? Time in front of a screen is time kids aren't active. See how much screen time kids of different ages get and tips for healthier activities.

AGE GROUP > 8-10 | 11-14 | 15-18

YOUTH AGES 15-18 SPEND ABOUT

7½ hours a day

IN FRONT OF A SCREEN USING ENTERTAINMENT MEDIA

NEARLY

4½

OF THESE ARE SPENT WATCHING TELEVISION

INSTEAD THEY COULD...

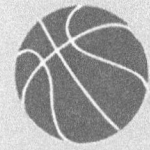

Play a game of basketball

AND STILL HAVE TIME TO...

walk the dog

and...

dance to their favorite songs

and...

go for a run

and...

do yard work

How can parents help?

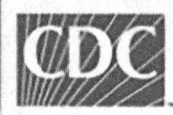

1 Ensure kids have 1 hour of physical activity each day.

2 Limit kids' total screen time to no more than 1–2 hours per day.

3 Remove TV sets from your child's bedroom.

4 Encourage other types of fun that include both physical and social activities, like joining a sports team or club.

FOR MORE INFORMATION, VISIT MakingHealthEasier.org/GetMoving

Resources:
American Academy of Pediatrics (AAP): Childhood obesity calls to action

Screen Time Policy Statement
CDC: Strategies to Prevent Obesity
Screen-Free Week

42. Which of the following is not a sign that the infographic is credible?

   A. The use of verifiable facts

   B. The list of source materials

   C. The professional appearance

   D. The inclusion of an author's name

43. Zetta is unsure of the credibility of this source and has never heard of the Centers for Disease Control (CDC). Which fact could help her decide to trust it?

   A. The CDC is located in Atlanta.

   B. The CDC has a .gov web address.

   C. The CDC creates many infographics.

   D. The CDC is also listed as a source consulted.

44. What could a skeptical reader do to verify the facts on the infographic?

   A. Interview one teenager to ask about his or her screen time

   B. Follow the links for the sources and determine their credibility

   C. Check a tertiary source like Wikipedia to verify the information

   D. Find different values for screen time on someone's personal blog

45. Which of the following would not be considered a credible source?

   A. Posts from social networks

   B. Materials published within the last 10 years

   C. Research articles written by respected and well-known authors

   D. Websites registered by government and educational institutions

Read both of the following texts and answer questions 46-53.

Passage 1:

Once when a Lion was asleep a little Mouse began running up and down upon him; this soon wakened the Lion, who placed his huge paw upon him, and opened his big jaws to swallow him. "Pardon, O King," cried the little Mouse: "forgive me this time, I shall never forget it: who knows but what I may be able to do you a turn some of these days?" The Lion was so tickled at the idea of the Mouse being able to help him, that he lifted up his paw and let him go. Sometime after the Lion was caught in a trap, and the hunters who desired to carry him alive to the King tied him to a tree while they went in search of a wagon to carry him on. Just then the little Mouse happened to pass by, and seeing the sad plight in which the Lion was, went up to him and soon gnawed away the ropes that bound the King of the Beasts. "Was I not right?" said the little Mouse.

Little friends may prove great friends.

Passage 2:

Beast left his mark on the fence.

It was lime green and slate gray and beautiful, so of course my father was outraged. If Beast hadn't had talent, Dad would have left it a while, but as it was, he got two of his parishioners to paint the thing over. Within the hour, the fence was back to being as white as the everlasting soul. My father's anger lasted longer than the tag.

The funny thing was, Beast loved my father. I don't know why. Life had knocked that kid down so hard so often he should have hated everything with the name of God stamped on it. But he loved my preacher father more than anyone else in the world. Maybe it was the dark suits and the white collars. Beast liked a pretty picture.

So there was my dad, ministering to the people in the worst parts of town, charging straight into drug dens and whorehouses to save people when they called him. He acted like he had no fear whatsoever. Plenty of the neighbors, the hardest-put ones, hated him for that. Lots of times he came close to getting his throat cut. More than once it was Beast who saved him.

And every time Beast saved my dad, he left his mark on the fence.

Dad couldn't stand it.

46. **What type of writing is used in the passages?**

    A. Both are narrative.

    B. Passage 1 is narrative and passage 2 is expository.

    C. Passage 1 is expository and passage 2 is narrative.

    D. Both are expository.

47. **Which term describes the structure of both passages?**

    A. Sequence

    B. Description

    C. Cause/effect

    D. Problem-solution

48. **Which statement accurately describes the genre of the passages?**

    A. Both are definitely fiction.

    B. Both are definitely nonfiction.

    C. Passage 1 is definitely nonfiction, and passage 2 is definitely fiction.

    D. Passage 1 is definitely fiction, and passage 2 could be fiction or nonfiction.

49. **Which label accurately describes the genre of passage 1?**

    A. Myth

    B. Fable

    C. Legend

    D. Mystery

50. **Which label could *not* accurately describe the genre of passage 2?**

    A. Legend

    B. Memoir

    C. Short story

    D. Autobiography

51. **Which statement describes a deeper meaning that is present in both passages?**

    A. Goodness comes out of evil deeds.

    B. In many ways, a preacher is like a lion.

    C. Help may come from unexpected sources.

    D. The biggest people are also the most violent.

52. **Which statement accurately describes a theme of passage 2?**

   A. All people, even evil ones, are mostly good.

   B. Street kids are good, and preachers are evil.

   C. There is a mixture of good and evil in everyone.

   D. Hypocrisy is the only truly evil trait a person can have.

53. **Which statement accurately describes how the two passages communicate their deeper meanings?**

   A. Both passages state implicit themes only.

   B. Both passages have an explicitly stated moral.

   C. Passage 1 states its point explicitly, and passage 2 states its point implicitly.

   D. Passage 1 states its point implicitly, and passage 2 states its point explicitly.

SECTION II. MATHEMATICS

You have 54 minutes to complete 36 questions.

1. The average person that weighs 150 pounds has approximately 4.5 liters of blood in their body. Based on that same scale, supposedly how many liters of blood would a 250-pound person have?

    A. 7.2 liters
    B. 6.75 liters
    C. 4.5 liters
    D. 7.5 liters

2. Write $1\frac{11}{20}$ as a percent.

    A. 150%
    B. 155%
    C. 200%
    D. 205%

3. If a company's revenue changes from $123 million to $118 million in a month, how quickly is it increasing in a year?

    A. −$60 million
    B. −$5 million
    C. $5 million
    D. $60 million

4. A circle has an area of 12 square feet. Find the diameter to the nearest tenth of a foot. Use 3.14 for π.

    A. 1.0
    B. 2.0
    C. 3.0
    D. 4.0

5. Convert 40 inches to millimeters. (Note: 1 inch is equal to 25.4 millimeters.)

    A. 101.6 millimeters
    B. 1,016 millimeters
    C. 10,160 millimeters
    D. 101,600 millimeters

6. A store has 75 pounds of bananas. Eight customers buy 3.3 pounds, five customers buy 4.25 pounds, and one customer buys 6.8 pounds. How many pounds are left in stock?

    A. 19.45
    B. 19.55
    C. 20.45
    D. 20.55

7. A rectangular garden needs a border. The length is $15\frac{3}{5}$ feet, and the width is $3\frac{2}{3}$ feet. What is the perimeter in feet?

    A. $18\frac{5}{8}$
    B. $19\frac{4}{15}$
    C. $37\frac{1}{4}$
    D. $38\frac{8}{15}$

8. Convert 15,000 grams to metric tons. (Note: 1 ton is equal to 1,000 kilograms and 1 kilogram is equal to 1,000 grams.)

    A. 0.00015 metric ton
    B. 0.0015 metric ton
    C. 0.015 metric ton
    D. 0.15 metric ton

9. A cubic storage bin has a volume of 216 cubic feet. What is the side length in feet? (Note: $V = s^3$.)

    A. 4
    B. 6
    C. 8
    D. 10

10. A man deposits $1,800 into a savings account that earns 8.3% annual interest. If he never adds any more money to the account, how much money will he have in a year?

    A. $1,949.40
    B. $1,494.00
    C. $2,240.90
    D. $1,994.40

11. A scientist wants his experimental fly population to grow by 100 flies every 3 days. If he starts with 300 flies, select the equation that represents how many he will have in one month (thirty days)?

    A. $100d + 300 = 1,300$ flies

    B. $\frac{300}{d} + 100 = 1,300$ flies

    C. $100\frac{d}{3} + 300 = 1,300$ flies

    D. $300d + 100 = 1,300$ flies

12. $2\frac{1}{2} \times 3\frac{3}{4}$

    A. $5\frac{3}{8}$ C. $7\frac{3}{8}$

    B. $6\frac{3}{8}$ D. $9\frac{3}{8}$

13. Write 62.42% as a fraction.

    A. $\frac{31}{50000}$ C. $\frac{3121}{50000}$

    B. $\frac{31}{5000}$ D. $\frac{3121}{5000}$

14. If 17 widgets failed but the other 1,273 worked properly, what is the failure rate of that widget?

    A. 1.30%   C. 1.34%

    B. 1.32%   D. 1.36%

15. Solve the equation for the unknown.

    $3x - 8 + 5 + 2x = 4x - x + 6$

    A. $-\frac{9}{2}$ C. $\frac{2}{9}$

    B. $-\frac{2}{9}$ D. $\frac{9}{2}$

16. The histogram below shows the amount a family spent on groceries during the year. Which statement is true for the histogram?

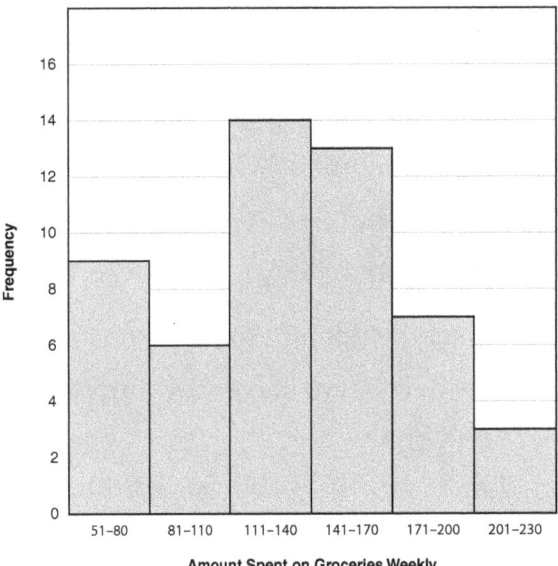

    A. The lowest frequency is between $80 and $110.

    B. The highest frequency is between $140 and $170.

    C. More than half of the amount spent is greater than $140.

    D. More than half of the amount spent is between $110 and $170.

17. **Find the values from the box plot.**

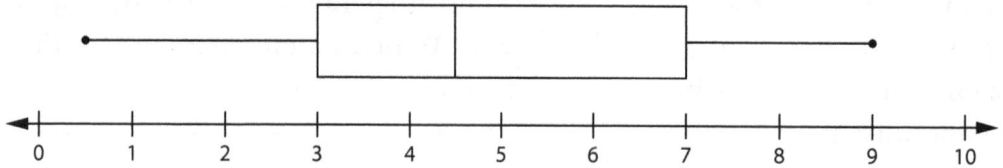

A. Minimum: 0, first quartile: 3, median: 5, third quartile: 7, maximum: 9

B. Minimum: 0.5, first quartile: 3, median: 4.5, third quartile: 7, maximum: 9

C. Minimum: 0, first quartile: 3, median: 5, third quartile: 7, maximum: 10

D. Minimum: 0.5, first quartile: 3, median: 4.5, third quartile: 7, maximum: 10

18. **Select the dot plot for the data below.**

The data below shows the number of minutes available to eat breakfast for a group of employees.

10, 20, 40, 30, 50, 60, 50, 40, 30, 20, 40, 30, 10, 20, 30, 50, 40, 10, 10, 20, 30, 40, 20, 50, 40, 30

A.   **Minutes to Eat Breakfast**   C.   **Minutes to Eat Breakfast**

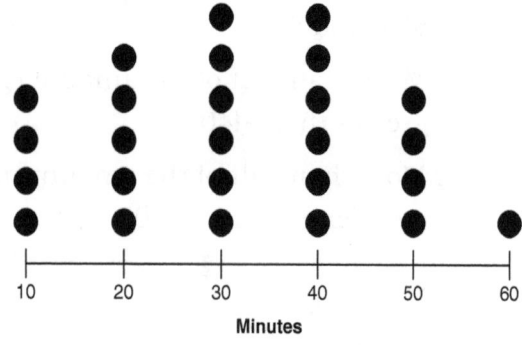

B.   **Minutes to Eat Breakfast**   D.   **Minutes to Eat Breakfast**

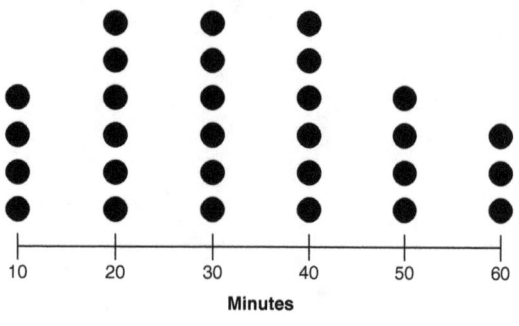

19. The line chart shows the number of cars sold each month. Which statement is true?

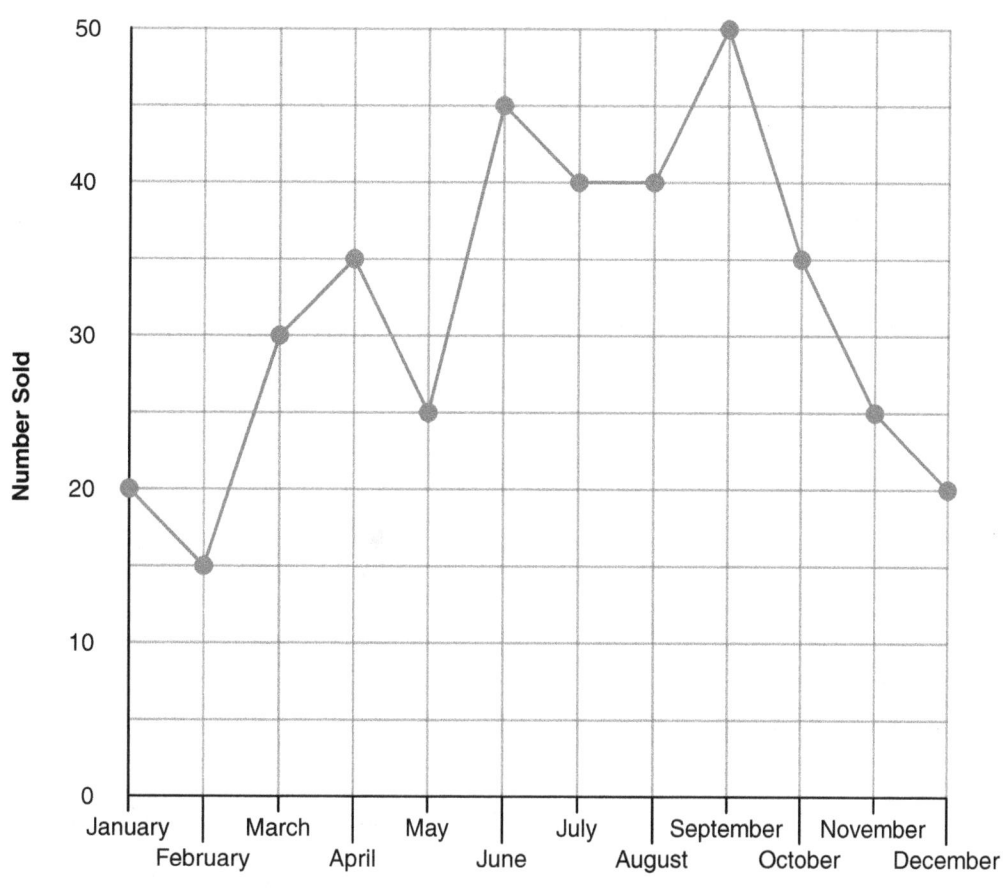

Cars Sold by Month

A. June had the most cars sold.

B. There were two months where 30 cars were sold.

C. The months with the smallest decreases all sold 5 fewer cars.

D. The difference between the highest and lowest month is 30 cars.

20. Solve the equation for the unknown.

$\frac{1}{2}x + 3 = \frac{1}{4}x - 2$

A. −20

B. −10

C. 10

D. 20

21. A server earns a 15% tip on average from the food he serves. If he serves $470 worth of food, how much money will he earn in tips?

A. $7.05

B. $70.50

C. $31.33

D. $10.57

17

22. The bar chart shows the number of items collected for a charity drive. What is the total number of items collected for the three highest classes?

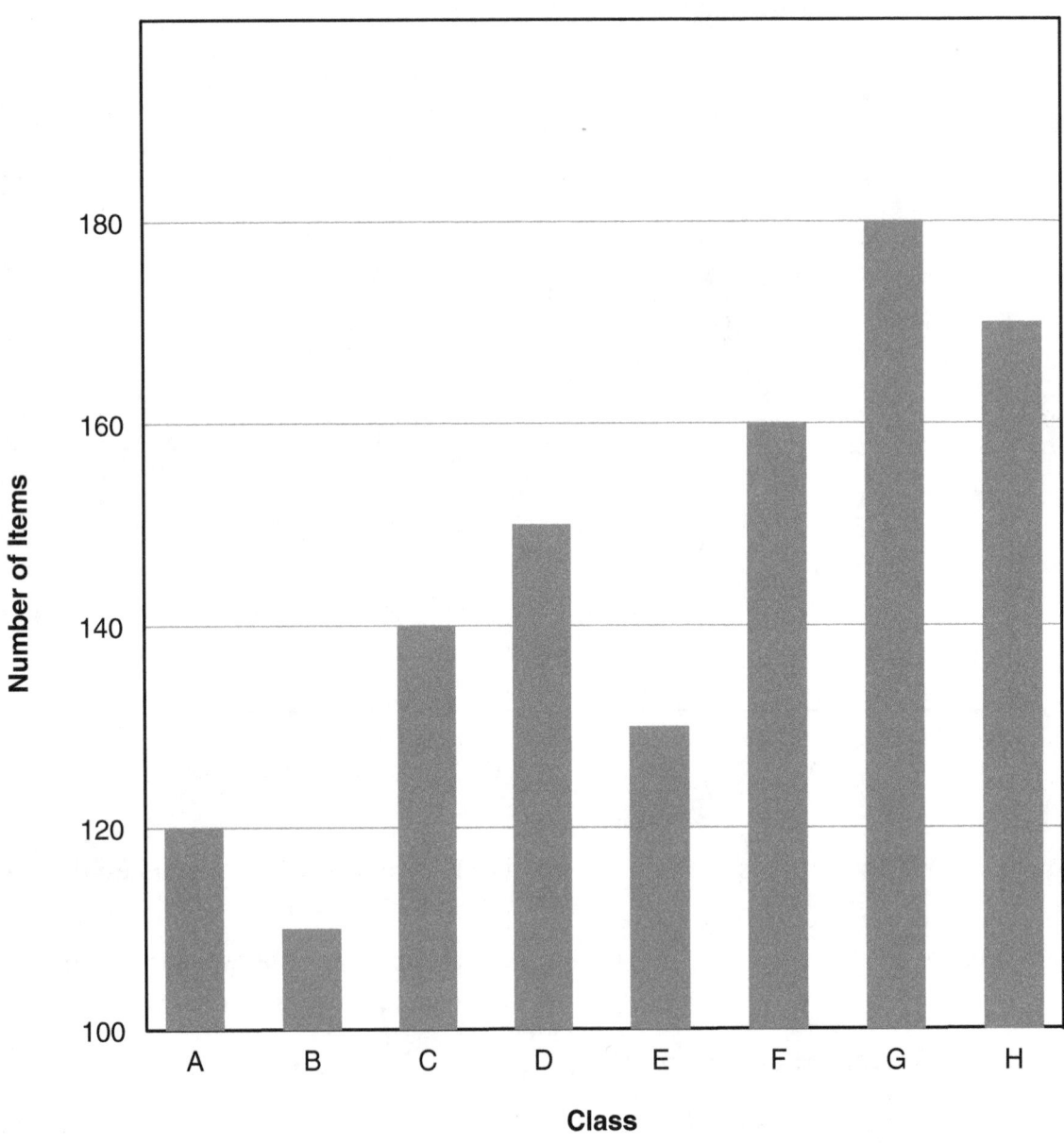

A. 500

B. 510

C. 520

D. 530

23. Hunter notices that she walked a total of 600 steps while walking around her work building on a 30-minute break. If she kept the same pace, how many steps could she walk if she took a 45-minute break?

A. 900
B. 750
C. 850
D. 800

24 What is 36% as a ratio?

A. 9:25
B. 36:100
C. 18:40
D. 25:9

25. Which is different from the others?

A. 6.4%
B. $\frac{8}{125}$
C. 128:2000
D. All of the above are equal.

26. Ross receives an employee discount of 12% at the furniture store he works for. If Ross selects $1,300 of merchandise, how much will he receive off his total with the discount?

A. $156
B. $1,284.40
C. $1,144
D. $15.60

27. $\frac{3}{8} + \frac{5}{6}$

A. $\frac{8}{14}$
B. $\frac{4}{7}$
C. $1\frac{1}{4}$
D. $1\frac{5}{24}$

28. A catering service provides small treats to a large corporate event. The service has an agreement to charge the hosting company only 85 cents per treat given at the event. If they serve 8 trays of 55 treats each, how much will the service bill be to the hosts?

A. $374
B. $440
C. $395
D. $415

29. $3\frac{1}{2} \div 2\frac{1}{2}$

A. $1\frac{1}{4}$
B. $1\frac{2}{5}$
C. $1\frac{1}{2}$
D. $1\frac{2}{3}$

30. $\frac{17}{12} + \frac{1}{4}$

A. $1\frac{1}{8}$
B. $1\frac{2}{3}$
C. $1\frac{1}{2}$
D. $1\frac{8}{15}$

31. A mechanic purchases 18 gallons of oil to complete a number of oil changes. If he needs $\frac{3}{10}$ a gallon of oil for each car, how many oil changes can he do before he runs out?

A. 54 oil changes
B. 60 oil changes
C. 15 oil changes
D. 34 oil changes

32. A photo center develops prints for $0.45 a photo. If their operations cost $3,100 a month in addition to 10 cents per photo, how many photos must they develop to see a $400 profit?

A. 6,000
B. 8,000
C. 10,000
D. 9,000

33. Solve the equation for the unknown x.

$y = mx + b$.

A. $y - bm = x$
B. $y + bm = x$
C. $\frac{y-b}{m} = x$
D. $\frac{y+b}{m} = x$

34. Perform the operation.

$(-3x + 5xy - 6y) - (4x + 2xy - 5y)$

A. $-7x + 7xy - y$
B. $-7x + 7xy - 11y$
C. $-7x + 3xy - y$
D. $-7x + 3xy - 11y$

35. A right triangle has a base of 6 inches
   and a hypotenuse of 10 inches. Find the
   height in inches of the triangle if the
   area is 24 square inches. (Note: $A = \frac{bh}{2}$.)

   A. 4   C. 8

   B. 6   D. 10

36. $1\frac{2}{3} \div 3\frac{7}{12}$

   A. $\frac{20}{43}$ C. $3\frac{3}{4}$

   B. $3\frac{7}{18}$ D. $5\frac{35}{36}$

SECTION III. SCIENCE

You have 63 minutes to complete 53 questions.

1. Which of the following cavities contains the urinary bladder, part of the intestines, and the internal reproductive organs?

   A. Abdominal   C. Pelvic

   B. Dorsal   D. Thoracic

2. Which plane of the body divides the body into two equal halves?

   A. Coronal   C. Sagittal

   B. Midsagittal   D. Transverse

3. Which of the following represents everything working optimally in a functioning human body?

   A. Diffusion   C. Metabolism

   B. Homeostasis   D. Variable

4. Which wave is associated with a ventricle systole?

   A. P wave   C. ST segment

   B. T wave   D. QRS complex

5. Which valve regulates blood flow between the right atrium and right ventricle?

   A. Aortic   C. Pulmonary

   B. Mitral   D. Tricuspid

6. Exchanges of substances like gases and nutrients occur at the

   A. arteries.

   B. capillaries.

   C. veins.

   D. venules.

7. What is a primary difference between intracellular chemical signals and intercellular chemical signals?

   A. Intercellular chemical signals produce rapid responses.

   B. Intracellular chemical signals produce rapid responses.

   C. Intercellular chemical signals produce electrical signals.

   D. Intracellular chemical signals produce electrical signals.

8. Which system secretes neurohormones?

   A. circulatory   C. integumentary

   B. digestive   D. nervous

9. Which of the following refers to the shape and chemical characteristics of each receptor site allowing only certain chemical signals to bind to it?

   A. Conductivity   C. Permeability

   B. Memory   D. Specificity

10. What is the most common cause of appendicitis?

   A. Spicy foods   C. An obstruction

   B. Poor nutrition   D. Inherited factor

11. What is the correct order of the sections of the large intestine as they lead to the rectum?

    A. Ascending, transverse, descending, and sigmoid

    B. Descending, transverse, ascending, and sigmoid

    C. Ascending, sigmoid, descending, and transverse

    D. Sigmoid, transverse, descending, and ascending

12. Which organ of the digestive system has villi?

    A. Pancreas   C. Large intestine

    B. Gallbladder   D. Small intestine

13. Which layer of the skin contains nerve endings?

    A. Dermis

    B. Epidermis

    C. Stratum basale

    D. Subcutaneous tissue

14. Which part of the skin is directly affected by the most common types of skin cancer?

    A. Dermis

    B. Epidermis

    C. Sebaceous glands

    D. Subcutaneous layer

15. Which of the following trigger the lymphatic system response against a pathogen without an infection occuring?

    A. B cells

    B. Antibodies

    C. Vaccinations

    D. Helper T cells

16. The B cells do not directly attack pathogens or infected cells. Instead, they

    A. mark the pathogens for destruction by macrophages and B cells.

    B. mark the antibodies for destruction by B cells and natural killer cells.

    C. mark the antibodies for destruction by macrophages and killer T cells.

    D. mark the pathogens for destruction by macrophages and natural killer cells.

17. What type of cells release histamines?

    A. B cells   C. Helper T cells

    B. Mast cells   D. Macrophage cells

18. Which of the following describes a cartilaginous joint?

    A. It is a type of immovable joint.

    B. It allows bones to be very flexible.

    C. It is the joint between vertebral discs of the spine.

    D. It operates as a hinge movement.

19. Muscles work together in a synchronized fashion through the action of:

    A. opening and closing.   C. stretching and pulling.

    B. moving up and down.   D. contracting and extending.

20. What muscle do circulating hormones stimulate?

    A. Extension   C. Skeletal

    B. Flexor   D. Smooth

21. Which of the following most likely directly stimulates the excitation of a neuron?

    A. Astrocyte

    B. Muscle fiber

    C. Myelin sheath

    D. Neurotransmitter

22. Nodes of Ranvier are

    A. spaces between myelin sheaths.

    B. cavities in the brain filled with fluid.

    C. dendrites that receive sensory inputs.

    D. chemical messages carried in vesicles.

23. Which of the following represents the divided, equal periods of time in a pregnancy?

    A. Trilogies

    B. Trimesters

    C. Semesters

    D. Menstrual cycles

24. Which statement about puberty is true?

    A. Puberty results from an unfertilized ovum.

    B. Males begin puberty at a younger age than females.

    C. Females begin puberty at a younger age than males.

    D. Puberty is a cyclical process occurring in the female body.

25. Which body system works with the respiratory system to aid in blood pH regulation?

    A. Digestive

    B. Integumentary

    C. Nervous

    D. Urinary

26. The oxygen concentration in blood that returns from systemic circulation is

    A. less than the oxygen concentration in the tissues.

    B. the same as the oxygen concentration in the tissues.

    C. more than the carbon dioxide concentration in the veins.

    D. the same as the carbon dioxide concentration in the veins.

27. Which organ, not belonging to the respiratory system, plays a direct role in external respiration?

    A. Heart

    B. Kidney

    C. Liver

    D. Stomach

28. Which of the following plays a role in bone tissue breakdown?

    A. Diaphysis

    B. Osteoclast

    C. Haversian canal

    D. Medullary cavity

29. What is a benefit of bone resorption?

    A. Releasing minerals into blood circulation

    B. Transforming soft tissue to hard connective tissue

    C. Creating avenues for nerve fibers to travel in bone

    D. Stimulating hematopoiesis for red blood cell development

30. What bone type is the patella classified as?

    A. Flat bone

    B. Long bone

    C. Short bone

    D. Sesamoid bone

31. The antidiuretic hormone ADH is known to alter the concentration of which of the following substances that is excreted from the urinary system?

    A. Ammonia
    B. Creatinine
    C. Sodium
    D. Urine

32. Where does fluid flow directly after leaving through the pores of Bowman's capsule?

    A. Bladder
    B. Glomerulus
    C. Loop of Henle
    D. Proximal convoluted tubule

33. Which is a classification level in the Linnaean system?

    A. Achaea
    B. Domain
    C. Genus
    D. Ursidae

34. Which is a characteristic of water?

    A. Nonpolarity
    B. Low boiling point
    C. Organic in nature
    D. Universal solvency

35. Which class of biomolecule helps transmit genetic information?

    A. Lipids
    B. Proteins
    C. Nucleic acids
    D. Carbohydrates

36. Which cell part stores waste material in the cell?

    A. Chloroplast
    B. Nucleus
    C. Ribosome
    D. Vacuole

37. What is a characteristic of eukaryotes?

    A. These organisms are all unicellular.
    B. They lack a membrane-bound nucleus.
    C. Many organelles are in their cytoplasm.
    D. Bacteria and plants are examples of eukaryotes.

38. Which is an example of a eukaryote?

    A. Archaea
    B. Bacteria
    C. Seaweed
    D. Virus

39. Why does photosynthesis need ATP?

    A. Make membranes
    B. Establish a gradient
    C. Produce chloroplasts
    D. Create sugar molecules

40. Which contains the most chlorophyll?

    A. Cyanobacteria
    B. Leaf
    C. Mushroom
    D. Prokaryote

41. Mitosis is different from meiosis because mitosis

    A. is a form of asexual reproduction.
    B. leads to the production of gametes.
    C. includes two rounds of cell division.
    D. results in increased genetic diversity.

42. If an organism has a total of 12 chromosomes, 12 is the _____ number of chromosomes.

    A. diploid
    B. equivalent
    C. haploid
    D. neutral

43. The DNA base cytosine only pairs with
_____.

A. adenine   C. guanine

B. cytosine   D. thymine

44. Why must researchers consider the placebo effect?

A. Monitor the outcome of the experiment

B. Ensure a proper independent variable is chosen

C. Account for the body's response to fake treatments

D. Create a baseline measure for experimental analysis

45. What is a treatment group?

A. A type of placebo

B. A baseline measure

C. The outcome of interest

D. The variable being manipulated

46. When a researcher determines the cause-and-effect relationship between two variables, what part of the scientific method is the researcher performing?

A. Analysis   C. Experiment

B. Conclusion   D. Hypothesis

47. Empirical evidence is

A. repeatable by multiple scientists.

B. used to explain the placebo effect.

C. created using deductive reasoning.

D. data that contains metric base units.

48. Which of the following describes one difference between the two most abundant isotopes of iron, iron-54 and iron-56?

A. Iron-56 has more protons than iron-54.

B. Iron-56 has more neutrons than iron-54.

C. Iron-54 and iron-56 have different atomic numbers.

D. Iron-54 and iron-56 contain different numbers of electrons.

49. Which of the following describes a neutral atom of tin-120?

A. 50 protons, 70 neutrons, 50 electrons

B. 50 protons, 120 neutrons, 50 electrons

C. 50 protons, 120 neutrons, 70 electrons

D. 70 protons, 120 neutrons, 70 electrons

50. In the chemical equation below, which element is unbalanced?

$$2HNO_3 + Na \rightarrow 2NaNO_3 + H_2$$

A. Hydrogen   C. Oxygen

B. Nitrogen   D. Sodium

51. What is a polar molecule?

A. A molecule that contains oxygen

B. A molecule that is repulsed by water

C. A molecule that is attracted to water

D. A molecule that has slight charges on each end

25

52. Net water movement through a membrane in response to the concentration of a solute is called _____.

    A. bonding   C. osmosis

    B. diffusion   D. polarity

53. In which of the following phases are particles of a substance generally closest together?

    A. Gas   C. Plasma

    B. Liquid   D. Solid

SECTION IV. ENGLISH AND LANGUAGE USAGE

You have 28 minutes to complete 28 questions.

1. **Which of the following is correct?**

    A. May

    B. Spring

    C. easter

    D. sunday

2. **Which sentence is incorrect?**

    A. I hate you!

    B. When does the movie start?

    C. I go to bed early so I do not feel tired.

    D. You should drink eight glasses of water a day.

3. **Which of the following spellings is correct?**

    A. Busines

    B. Business

    C. Buseness

    D. Bussiness

4. **Which of the following words correctly completes the following sentence?**

    It was a treacherous route, and they traveled more _____ when they had a guide.

    A. safe

    B. safer

    C. safest

    D. safely

5. **Which word is not a conjunction?**

    A. Or

    B. The

    C. So

    D. But

6. **Which of the following nouns can be made plural by simply adding -*s*?**

    A. Fox

    B. Frog

    C. Cherry

    D. Potato

7. **Which word in the following sentence is a pronoun?**

    To whom should the applicant address the letter?

    A. To

    B. the

    C. whom

    D. should

8. **Which part of the following sentence is the predicate?**

    Mai and her friend Oksana love to ride roller coasters.

    A. Mai and her friend Oksana

    B. and her friend Oksana

    C. love to ride roller coasters

    D. roller coasters

9. **Which of the following subjects correctly agrees with the verb "Watch" in this sentence?**

    <u>Watch</u> out!

    A. You

    B. He

    C. I

    D. Out

10. **Which word in the following sentence is a helping verb?**

    They did not ask for our help.

    A. did

    B. ask

    C. for

    D. our

11. **Fill in the blank with the correct subordinating conjunction.**

    You cannot go to the movies with your friends _____ you finish your homework.

    A. if

    B. once

    C. since

    D. unless

12. **Fill in the blank with the correct subordinating conjunction.**

    I had a bad stomach flu but started to regain my appetite, _____ is good news.

    A. so
    B. that
    C. which
    D. whereas

13. **Fill in the blank with the correct coordinating conjunction.**

    Desert climates are hot and dry, _____ many plants grow there.

    A. so
    B. yet
    C. for
    D. and

14. **Which of the following is an example of a compound sentence?**

    A. The Jankowskis typically go out for Italian food, tonight they tried Thai.
    B. The Jankowskis typically go out for Italian food and tonight they tried Thai.
    C. The Jankowskis typically go out for Italian food, but tonight they tried Thai.
    D. The Jankowskis typically go out for Italian food even though tonight they tried Thai.

15. **Which of the following options would complete the sentence below to make it a simple sentence?**

    You can see the wonders of our country _____

    A. on a road trip.
    B. take a road trip.
    C. and, on a road trip.
    D. rather than taking a road trip.

16. **Which of the following sentences uses the MOST informal language?**

    A. I must go to school.
    B. I have to go to school.
    C. I need to go to school.
    D. I gotta go to school.

17. **Which of the following sentences uses the MOST formal language?**

    A. Congrats!
    B. Congratulations!
    C. Congratulations on your recent success.
    D. Congrats to you.

18. **Which of the following sentences uses the MOST informal language?**

    A. The house creaked at night.
    B. I ate dinner with my friend.
    C. It's sort of a bad time.
    D. The water trickled slowly.

19. **Which of the following is the meaning of "bolt" as used in this sentence?**

    When the young boy saw his angry mother coming toward him, he made a bolt for the door.

    A. A large roll of cloth
    B. A quick movement in a particular direction
    C. A sliding bar that is used to lock a window or door
    D. A bright line of light appearing in the sky during a storm

20. Which of the following context clues correctly helps you define the word "bind" in this sentence?

The mayonnaise is the key ingredient that will <u>bind</u> the egg salad together.

A. "key"
B. "ingredient"
C. "salad"
D. "together"

21. Which of the following context clues correctly helps you define the word "emulate" in this sentence?

Felicia always tried to <u>emulate</u> her big sister, so she would often imitate the way she spoke, moved, and how she dressed.

A. "tried"
B. "often"
C. "imitate "
D. "way"

22. Which of the following is the meaning of "novice" as used in this sentence?

Since he was a <u>novice</u> at playing chess, he took lessons with a master to get more experience.

A. Failure
B. Natural
C. Teacher
D. Beginner

23. Which of the following words in this sentence has more than one meaning?

Candace and her brother love to play in the leaves.

A. brother
B. love
C. play
D. leaves

24. Which of the following suffixes means "in a manner of or resembling"?

A. -ful
B. -able
C. -less
D. -esque

25. Which of the following root words means people?

A. ject
B. fasc
C. dem
D. cycl

26. Which of the following prefixes means "former"?

A. ex-
B. de-
C. in-
D. sub-

27. The use of the prefix *mono-* in the word *monolingual* indicates that a person knows which of the following about language?

A. How to teach a language
B. How to speak one language
C. How to learn a language quickly
D. How to speak several languages

28. *Bilateral* most nearly means

A. affecting one area.
B. relating to two sides.
C. pertaining to the inside of.
D. referring to the entire being.

TEAS PRACTICE EXAM 1
ANSWER KEY WITH EXPLANATORY ANSWERS

Section I. Reading

1. B. The second sentence of this paragraph expresses the main idea that chocolate chip cookies were invented by accident. This makes it the topic sentence. **Skill: Main Ideas, Topic Sentences, and Supporting Details.**

2. A. The topic of a sentence is a word or phrase that describes what the text is about. **Skill: Main Ideas, Topic Sentences, and Supporting Details.**

3. C. This paragraph presents the story behind the invention of the chocolate chip cookie. It discusses the fact that the dessert was a complete accident. This idea is expressed in a topic sentence at the beginning of the paragraph. **Skill: Main Ideas, Topic Sentences, and Supporting Details.**

4. D. The main idea of this paragraph is that chocolate chip cookies were invented by accident. The detail that directly supports this is the one describing what Ruth Graves Wakefield did when she ran out of baker's chocolate – she broke up a block of Nestle semi-sweet chocolate expecting them to melt. This is a supporting detail. **Skill: Main Ideas, Topic Sentences, and Supporting Details.**

5. B. All of the above sentences relate to the topic of chocolate chip cookies, but only the sentence about Ruth Graves Wakefield realizing how delicious they were relates directly to the main idea that the chocolate chip cookie was invented by accident. **Skill: Main Ideas, Topic Sentences, and Supporting Details.**

6. B. This paragraph discusses the past and future in a way that shifts constantly between the two. Some events are vague and may overlap with others. However, coming to America is a clear event that happened before the escape from physical poverty and the entrance into the poverty of the soul. **Skill: Summarizing Text and Using Text Features.**

7. B. This summary is effective because it restates only the key points and it does it using new words. **Skill: Summarizing Text and Using Text Features.**

8. A. An ineffective summary would copy the original text word for word and only change one or two words. The first sentence is almost exactly like the first sentence of the original text, so this would be structurally plagiarized. **Skill: Summarizing Text and Using Text Features.**

9. D. A summary that is structurally plagiarized would be ineffective since it would involve rewriting the original words one by one and only changing a few of them. **Skill: Summarizing Text and Using Text Features.**

10. B. If this paragraph were organized more sequentially, it would feel less scattered. Putting on gloves comes before the other actions, so it would be best to place sentence 5 before sentence 2. **Skill: The Writing Process.**

11. A. Working slowly and loosening the plug happen at the same time. The active and grammatically correct way to express this is, "Using your wrench, slowly loosen the plug." **Skill: The Writing Process.**

12. C. The sentence explains why it's a good idea to keep your hands away from the stream. It would work best after sentence 4. **Skill: The Writing Process.**

13. D. Revision isn't just fixing errors; it's the process of strengthening content and organization in writing. **Skill: Essay Revision and Transitions.**

14. C. Referring vaguely to "a study" is not particularly trustworthy because it does not allow the reader a chance to verify the information or the credentials of the authors. Naming the study and its authors could eliminate this problem. **Skill: Essay Revision and Transitions.**

15. D. The evidence does not clearly support the statement that a 7:15 a.m. start time is damaging to students. It does show that some teenagers may not learn optimally if they are following their bodies' tendency to stay up later than adults. **Skill: Essay Revision and Transitions.**

16. B. The final sentence of this paragraph attacks the people who disagree with the author's point. This manipulative use of the emotions weakens the overall argument. **Skill: Essay Revision and Transitions.**

17. D. The transition is the word that links the two ideas: *thereafter*. This word doesn't appear between the two sentences, but it does show how the two sentences are related in time. **Skill: Tone, Mood, and Transition Words.**

18. A. Transition words like "however" express a contrast between ideas. **Skill: Tone, Mood, and Transition Words.**

19. D. The tone of this letter is appreciative as the author openly thanks the teacher for all he has done for her daughter. **Skill: Tone, Mood, and Transition Words.**

20. D. The author of the letter uses a lot of respectful and admiring language, but the line "We cannot thank you enough" has an especially appreciative and warm tone. **Skill: Tone, Mood, and Transition Words.**

21. B. A teacher receiving a note like this would likely feel grateful. **Skill: Tone, Mood, and Transition Words.**

22. D. The phrase "above all" adds emphasis to the writer's point that the teacher has made a significant impact on the daughter. **Skill: Tone, Mood, and Transition Words.**

23. B. An author's purpose is his or her reason for writing. **Skill: Understanding Author's Purpose, Point of View, and Rhetorical Strategies.**

24. C. This is an advertisement. Although it includes some information its primary purpose is to convince you to buy something. This makes it a persuasive text. **Skill: Understanding the Author's Purpose, Point of View, and Rhetorical Strategies.**

25. D. Writers of advertisements are tasked with selling a product; therefore, it is difficult to know much about their true feelings. However, it is a fair bet that advertising writers believe people will pay money for products presented the way they describe. **Skill: Understanding the Author's Purpose, Point of View, and Rhetorical Strategies.**

26. C. Much of the information in this advertisement is not verifiable, but the fact that the Wizard WiFi contains functions to set and track family usage is verifiable. **Skill: Understanding the Author's Purpose, Point of View, and Rhetorical Strategies.**

27. C. The advertisement highlights several aspects of Wizard WiFi's functionality, such as ease of use, that suggest the potential customer will feel good using the products. These details appeal to the emotions. **Skill: Understanding the Author's Purpose, Point of View, and Rhetorical Strategies.**

28. D. Celebrity endorsements in advertisements appeal to the emotions by associating a product for sale with a person who is widely admired. **Skill: Understanding the Author's Purpose, Point of View, and Rhetorical Strategies.**

29. B. Formatting features make text stand out in a title or within a paragraph. Charts are graphic elements that present data or illustrate information. **Skill: Evaluating and Integrating Data.**

30. C. An argument may include both verifiably true statements, or facts, and statements based on belief, or opinions. **Skill: Facts, Opinions, and Evaluating an Argument.**

31. B. Writers can eliminate gender bias by repeating a title rather than using a pronoun. **Skill: Facts, Opinions, and Evaluating an Argument.**

32. D. An article on the best farming practices from the turn of the 19th century would be highly outdated. Even if the writer were a professional farmer, the advice presented would likely not be worth following. **Skill: Understanding Primary Sources, Making Inferences, and Drawing Conclusions.**

33. C. The label shows the number of calories per serving: 150. **Skill: Evaluating and Integrating Data.**

34. B. The label shows that there are 20 calories per serving. 60 crackers would be three servings. **Skill: Evaluating and Integrating Data.**

35. D. Although the sodium content is not low, only the saturated fat value is considered particularly high. **Skill: Evaluating and Integrating Data.**

36. A. Products are considered low in a nutrient if the Daily Value is below 5%. This product does not meet that criterion. **Skill: Evaluating and Integrating Data.**

37. A. Although this product would not be considered healthy by most standards, it is a good source of iron. **Skill: Evaluating and Integrating Data.**

38. A. The argument that getting rid of homework is undoubtedly beneficial is an opinion statement because it makes a judgment. **Skill: Facts, Opinions, and Evaluating an Argument.**

39. C. The statement is a fact because it discusses the results of standardized test scores, which can be measured. **Skill: Facts, Opinions, and Evaluating an Argument.**

40. B. The main argument in this passage is that there are no clear benefits from giving elementary-aged students daily homework. **Skill: Facts, Opinions, and Evaluating an Argument.**

41. D. The sentence about homework doing nothing to enhance student learning at all is an overgeneralization. The term "at all" makes a big over-arching claim that cannot be verified, as the author does not even explore some of the potential benefits of daily homework. **Skill: Facts, Opinions, and Evaluating an Argument.**

42. C. The appearance of this infographic has to do with its design, not its content. Therefore, the professional appearance of an infographic is not an indication that the content is credible. It is usually a good sign if an author is clearly named in a source. Although this source is authored by an organization, the CDC, which is a well-known organization with a good reputation, instead of a single author, there are many other signs it is credible. **Skill: Understanding Primary Sources, Making Inferences, and Drawing Conclusions.**

43. B. When presenting this type of information, a government organization with a .gov web address is typically considered a reputable source. **Skill: Understanding Primary Sources, Making Inferences, and Drawing Conclusions.**

44. B. One way to verify facts is to check the sources an author used. Verifying facts elsewhere may also be a good idea, but it is important to use reputable primary or secondary sources. **Skill: Understanding Primary Sources, Making Inferences, and Drawing Conclusions.**

45. A. Posts from social media networks, such as Facebook, are not considered to be credible sources because they contain an individual's opinion and cannot be verified as factual. **Skill: Understanding Primary Sources, Making Inferences, and Drawing Conclusions.**

46. A. Both passages tell stories. That makes this narrative writing. **Skill: Types of Passages, Text Structures, Genre and Theme.**

47. A. Both passages say what happened first, second, third, and so on, in chronological order. This is a sequential structure. **Skill: Types of Passages, Text Structures, Genre and Theme.**

48. D. Passage 1, with its talking animal characters, is definitely fiction. Passage 2 could be nonfiction (memoir or autobiography) or fiction (short story or novel). **Skill: Types of Passages, Text Structures, Genre and Theme.**

49. B. Passage 1 is a short fantastical tale for children that teaches an explicit lesson. This makes it a fable. **Skill: Types of Passages, Text Structures, Genre and Theme.**

50. A. Passage 2 could be a novel excerpt, a short story, or a section from an autobiography or memoir. It is least likely to be a legend. **Skill: Types of Passages, Text Structures, Genre and Theme.**

51. C. In passage 1, the mouse helps a lion, and in passage 2, a street kid helps a priest. In both passages, help comes from an unexpected source. **Skill: Types of Passages, Text Structures, Genre and Theme.**

52. C. Passage 2 seems concerned with good and evil and people's expectations of both, but it doesn't clearly point to a message about who is evil or which traits are worse than others. The two people it describes are both flawed but capable of doing good, so one theme may be that everyone contains a mixture of both good and evil. **Skill: Types of Passages, Text Structures, Genre and Theme.**

53. C. Passage 1 is a fable with an explicitly stated moral: "Little friends may prove great friends." Passage 2 has more subtle themes that are both implicit and harder to define. **Skill: Types of Passages, Text Structures, Genre and Theme.**

Section II. Mathematics

1. D. A 250-pound person would supposedly have 7.5 liters becaus $\frac{4.5 \text{ liters}}{150 \text{ pounds}} = \frac{X}{250 \text{ pounds}}$ and $X = 7.5$ liters of blood. **Skill: Ratios, Proportions, and Percentages.**

2. B. The correct answer is 155% because $1\frac{11}{20}$ as a percent is $1.55 \times 100 = 155\%$. **Skill: Decimals and Fractions.**

3. A. The company's revenue is decreasing −$60 million in a year. Begin by calculating the revenue decrease, which is the difference between $118 million and $123 million, or −$5 million. That decrease is for one month. Next, set up a proportion to find the equivalent rate of change for a year, noting that a year is 12 months:

$$\frac{-\$5 \text{ million}}{1 \text{ month}} = \frac{?}{12 \text{ months}}$$

Because the denominator on the right is 12 times the denominator on the left, find the unknown rate of change by multiplying −$5 million by 12 to get −$60 million. Because the question asked for a rate of increase but the revenue is decreasing, the negative sign is critical. **Skill: Ratios, Proportions, and Percentages.**

4. D. The correct solution is 4.0 because $A = \pi r^2$; $12 = 3.14\, r^2$; $3.82 = r^2$; $r \approx 2.0$. The diameter is twice the radius, or about 4.0 feet. **Skill: Circles.**

5. B. The correct solution is 1,016 millimeters. 40 in. $\times \frac{2.54\ \text{cm}}{1\ \text{in.}} \times \frac{10\ \text{mm}}{1\ \text{cm}} = 1{,}016$ mm. **Skill: Standards of Measure.**

6. D. The correct solution is 20.55 because the number of pounds purchased is $8(3.3) + 5(4.25) + 6.8 = 26.4 + 21.25 + 6.8 = 54.45$ pounds. The number of pounds remaining is 75–54.45 = 20.55 pounds. **Skill: Solving Real World Mathematical Problems.**

7. D. The correct solution is $38\frac{8}{15}$ because $15\frac{3}{5} + 3\frac{2}{3} = 15\frac{9}{15} + 3\frac{10}{15} = 18\frac{19}{15}(2) = \frac{289}{15} \times \frac{2}{1} = \frac{578}{15} = 38\frac{8}{15}$ feet. **Skill: Solving Real World Mathematical Problems.**

8. C. The correct solution is 0.015 metric ton. $15{,}000\ \text{g} \times \frac{1\ \text{kg}}{1{,}000\ \text{g}} \times \frac{1\ \text{t}}{1{,}000\ \text{kg}} = \frac{15{,}000}{1{,}000{,}000} = 0.015$ t. **Skill: Standards of Measure.**

9. B. The correct solution is 6. Substitute the values into the formula, $216 = s^3$. Apply the cube root to both sides of the equation, $s = 6$ feet. **Skill: Similarity, Right Triangles, and Trigonometry.**

10. A. The man will have $1,949.40 because the annual interest will earn him $149.40. $1,800 $\times$ 0.083 = $149.40 + $1,800 = $1,949.40. **Skill: Ratios, Proportions, and Percentages.**

11. C. The equation is $100\frac{d}{3} + 300 = 1{,}300$ flies because the scientist should have 1,300 flies. In thirty days, the population will have hopefully gone through 10 growth cycles, so the multiplier is the number of days divided by 3. If each growth cycle increases the fly population by 100, the scientist will have an additional 1,000 flies. **Skill: Ratios, Proportions, and Percentages.**

12. D. The correct solution is $9\frac{3}{8}$ because $\frac{5}{2} \times \frac{15}{4} = \frac{75}{8} = 9\frac{3}{8}$. **Skill: Multiplication and Division of Fractions.**

13. D. The correct answer is $\frac{3121}{5000}$ because 62.42% as a fraction is $\frac{6242}{10000} = \frac{3121}{5000}$. **Skill: Decimals and Fractions.**

14. B. The failure rate is 1.32%. The failure rate is the fraction of all widgets that failed. In this case, the total number of widgets is 17 + 1,273 = 1,290. The failure rate is therefore $\frac{17}{1290}$, which is about 1.32%. **Skill: Ratios, Proportions, and Percentages.**

15. D. The correct solution is $\frac{9}{2}$. **Skill: Equations with One Variable.**

$5x–3 = 3x + 6$	Combine like terms on the left and right sides of the equation.
$2x–3 = 6$	Subtract $3x$ from both sides of the equation.
$2x = 9$	Add 3 to both sides of the equation.
$x = \frac{9}{2}$	Divide both sides of the equation by 2.

16. D. The correct solution is more than half of the amount spent is between $110 and $170. There are 14 weeks where the amount spent is between $110 and $140 and 13 weeks where the amount spent is between $140 and $170. This is 27 weeks, which is more than half the data set. **Skill: Interpreting Categorical and Quantitative Data.**

17. B. The correct solution is minimum: 0.5, first quartile: 3, median: 4.5, third quartile: 7, maximum: 9, which are the values of the box plot. **Skill: Interpreting Categorical and Quantitative Data.**

18. A. The correct solution is A. There are 4 employees who have 10 minutes and 50 minutes, 5 employees who have 20 minutes, 6 employees who have 30 minutes and 40 minutes, and 1 employee who has 60 minutes. **Skill: Interpreting Categorical and Quantitative Data.**

19. C. The correct solution is the months with the smallest decreases all sold 5 fewer cars. There was a decline of 5 cars from January to February, June to July, and from November to December. **Skill: Interpreting Graphics.**

20. A. The correct solution is −20.

$2x + 12 = x–8$	Multiply all terms by the least common denominator of 4 to eliminate the fractions.
$x + 12 = –8$	Subtract x from both sides of the equation.
$x = –20$	Subtract 12 from both sides of the equation.

Skill: Equations with One Variable.

21. B. The server will earn $70.50 in tips because $470 × 0.15 = $70.50. **Skill: Ratios, Proportions, and Percentages.**

22. B. The correct solution is 510 items because the three largest classes collected 180, 170, and 160 items. **Skill: Interpreting Graphics.**

23. A. Hunter could walk 900 steps in 45 minutes because $\frac{600 \text{ steps}}{30 \text{ minutes}} = \frac{X}{45 \text{ minutes}}$ and X = 900 steps. **Skill: Ratios, Proportions, and Percentages.**

24. A. As a ratio, 36% is 9:25. The most direct route is to convert 36% to a fraction, $\frac{36}{100}$, then reduce to lowest terms: $\frac{9}{25}$. The equivalent ratio in colon notation is 9:25. **Skill: Ratios, Proportions, and Percentages.**

25. D. All of the answer choices are equal. Although answer C is not in lowest terms, it is equal to $\frac{8}{125}$, which is equal to 0.064 or 6.4%. **Skill: Ratios, Proportions, and Percentages.**

26. A. Ross received $156 off of his $1300 total. Converting 12% to a decimal, 0.12 × $1,300 = $156. **Skill: Ratios, Proportions, and Percentages.**

27. D. The correct solution is $1\frac{5}{24}$ because $\frac{3}{8} + \frac{5}{6} = \frac{9}{24} + \frac{20}{24} = \frac{29}{24} = 1\frac{5}{24}$. **Skill: Addition and Subtraction of Fractions.**

28. A. The bill will be \$374 because 8×55 = 440 treats × \$0.85 = \$374. **Skill: Solving Real World Mathematical Problems.**

29. B. The correct answer is $1\frac{2}{5}$ because $\frac{7}{2} \div \frac{5}{2} = \frac{7}{2} \times \frac{2}{5} = \frac{14}{10} = 1\frac{4}{10} = 1\frac{2}{5}$. **Skill: Multiplication and Division of Fractions.**

30. B. The correct solution is $1\frac{2}{3}$ because $\frac{17}{12} + \frac{1}{4} = \frac{17}{12} + \frac{3}{12} = \frac{17+3}{12} = \frac{20}{12} = 1\frac{8}{12} = 1\frac{2}{3}$. **Skill: Addition and Subtraction of Fractions.**

31. B. The mechanic can do 60 oil changes because 18 gallons ÷ 0.3 gallons per car = 60 oil changes. **Skill: Solving Real World Mathematical Problems.**

32. C. The shop must sell 10,000 photos because they earn a 35 cent profit off each one printed. \$3,100 + \$400 = \$3,500 total ÷ \$0.35 profit = 10,000 photos. **Skill: Solving Real World Mathematical Problems.**

33. C. The correct solution is $\frac{y-b}{m} = x$.

$y - b = mx$ Subtract b from both sides of the equation.

$\frac{y-b}{m} = x$ Divide both sides of the equation by m.

Skill: Equations with One Variable.

34. C. The correct solution is $-7x + 3xy - y$.

$(-3x + 5xy - 6y) - (4x + 2xy - 5y) = (-3x + 5xy - 6y) + (-4x - 2xy + 5y)$
$= (-3x - 4x) + (5xy - 2xy) + (-6y + 5y) = -7x + 3xy - y$

Skill: Polynomials.

35. C. The correct solution is 8. Substitute the values into the formula, $24 = \frac{1}{2}(6)h$ and simplify the right side of the equation, $24 = 3h$. Divide both sides of the equation by 3, $h = 8$ inches. **Skill: Similarity, Right Triangles, and Trigonometry.**

36. A. The correct answer is $\frac{20}{43}$ because $\frac{5}{3} \div \frac{43}{12} = \frac{5}{3} \times \frac{12}{43} = \frac{60}{129} = \frac{20}{43}$. **Skill: Multiplication and Division of Fractions.**

Section III. Science

1. C. The pelvic cavity is a small space enclosed by the bones of the pelvis that contains the urinary bladder, part of the intestines, and the internal reproductive organs. **Skill: Organization of the Human Body.**

2. B. The midsagittal plane divides the body into two equal parts. **Skill: Organization of the Human Body.**

3. B. Homeostasis is the steady, optimal condition of a human body. **Skill: Organization of the Human Body.**

4. D. When a ventricular systole occurs, the ventricle is contracting. This is associated with the QRS complex on the electrocardiogram. **Skill: Cardiovascular System.**

5. D. As blood flows out of the right atrium into the right ventricle, the tricuspid valve prevents blood from flowing back into the right atrium. **Skill: Cardiovascular System.**

6. B. Classified as the thinnest blood vessels with the largest surface areas, the struture of capillaries facilitates exchanges of substances between blood and body tissues. **Skill: Cardiovascular System.**

7. A. Intercellular chemical signals that bind to membrane-bound receptors produce rapid responses. **Skill: Endocrine System.**

8. D. Neurohormones are secreted by the nervous system. **Skill: Endocrine System.**

9. D. Specificity is the characteristic that causes chemical signals to connect only to the correct receptors. **Skill: Endocrine System.**

10. C. The most common cause of appendicitis is an obstruction. **Skill: Gastrointestinal System.**

11. A. The correct sequence of the four parts of the large intestine is ascending, transverse, descending, and sigmoid. **Skill: Gastrointestinal System.**

12. D. The small intestine has finger-like projections called villi covering the internal surface. **Skill: Gastrointestinal System.**

13. A. The skin is comprised of three layers: epidermis, dermis, and subcutaneous tissue layer. The epidermis is the outermost layer and does not contain nerve endings. The dermis is the middle layer of skin that contains nerve endings. **Skill: Integumentary System.**

14. B. Basal cell carcinoma affects basal cells in the epidermis, while squamous cell carcinoma affects keratinocytes in the epidermis. Malignant melanoma affects melanocytes in the epidermis. **Skill: Integumentary System.**

15. C. Vaccinations trigger the lymphatic system response against a pathogen without an infection occurring. **Skill: The Lymphatic System.**

16. D. The B cells do not directly attack pathogens or infected cells. Instead, they mark the pathogens for destruction by macrophages and natural killer cells. When a B cell encounters a foreign microbe with a surface protein that matches the shape of its antibodies, it attaches an antibody to the microbe. **Skill: The Lymphatic System.**

17. B. The inflammatory response begins when mast cells release histamines and other chemicals that cause capillaries to swell. **Skill: The Lymphatic System.**

18. C. There are three types of joints in the human body: synovial, immovable, and partly movable. Partly moveable joints are also called cartilaginous joints. Cartilaginous joints hold bones together entirely by cartilage, allowing more movement between bones than a fibrous joint but less than the synovial joint. There are two main types of cartilaginous joints: synchondroses (primary cartilaginous) and symphyses (secondary cartilaginous). Examples of synchodroses cartilaginous joints include: epiphyseal growth plates in children, and between the sternum and first rib. Symphyses (held together by fibrocartilage) joints include: the pubic symphysis, and in the vertebral discs of the spine. **Skill: Muscular System.**

19. D. All muscles have the ability to contract and extend. To work together, all muscles contract (or shorten) and extend (or lengthen) in pairs following stimulation from the nervous system. **Skill: Muscular System.**

20. D. Either the nervous system or circulating hormones stimulate smooth muscle. This muscle is under involuntary control through both forms of stimulation. **Skill: Muscular System.**

21. D. A neurotransmitter is a type of substance that is released from the presynaptic membrane of one neuron and binds to the receptor on the postsynaptic membrane of a different neuron. By binding, this substance stimulates excitation of the neuron causing a neural impulse to be transmitted. **Skill: The Nervous System.**

22. A. Nodes of Ranvier are the gaps in myelin sheaths that increase the speed of an electrical neural signal down the axon of a neuron. **Skill: The Nervous System.**

23. B. Pregnancy typically lasts for about 40 weeks, which are traditionally divided into three periods of about 13 weeks each called trimesters. **Skill: Reproductive System.**

24. C. Females generally begin puberty at 10–11 years old; males generally begin puberty about a year later, at 11–12 years old. **Skill: Reproductive System.**

25. C. The nervous and cardiovascular systems work with the respiratory system to regulate blood pH levels. **Skill: The Respiratory System.**

26. A. After gas exchange occurs between blood and cells in body tissues, oxygen-poor blood travels in systemic circulation back to the heart and lungs. This blood has less oxygen and more carbon dioxide. Because oxygen diffuses into the tissues to the cells, oxygen concentration is higher in the tissues than in blood that returns to the heart via the veins. **Skill: The Respiratory System.**

27. A. The heart belongs to the cardiovascular system. It pumps oxygenated blood through systemic circulation and transports deoxygenated blood back to the lungs. **Skill: The Respiratory System.**

28. B. Osteoclasts are bone cells that play a role in bone remodeling. They are found on the surface of bone and aid in bone breakdown by dissolving worn-out bone tissue. **Skill: Skeletal System.**

29. A. Bone resorption is a process that dissolves old bone tissue so that it can undergo remodeling to produce new bone tissue. When bones dissolve during the resorption process, minerals stored in reservoirs of bone are released and pushed through circulation for use. **Skill: Skeletal System.**

30. D. Sesamoid bone consists of small bones like the patella. These bones provide mechanical support and protection. **Skill: Skeletal System.**

31. D. The posterior pituitary gland at the base of the brain secretes the hormone ADH. This hormone alters how much water is excreted from urine by the kidneys. Thus, it controls the concentration and volume of urine in the body. **Skill: The Urinary System.**

32. D. After filtered fluid leaves Bowman's capsule, which encloses the glomerulus, it travels to the proximal convoluted tubule before ending up in the loop of Henle. **Skill: The Urinary System.**

33. C. There are seven classification systems in the classical Linnaean system: kingdom, phylum, class, order, family, genus, and species. **Skill: An Introduction to Biology.**

34. D. Water is an excellent solvent that has the ability to dissolve many different substances and participate in a wide range of biochemical reactions. **Skill: An Introduction to Biology.**

35. C. Nucleic acids such as DNA and RNA are a class of biomolecules that play a role in the transmission of genetic information. **Skill: An Introduction to Biology.**

36. D. Found in both plant and animal cells, a vacuole functions as a storage site for many substances in the cell. **Skill: Cell Structure, Function, and Type.**

37. C. Eukaryotic cells are unicellular or multicellular organisms that contain a membrane-bound nucleus. Eukaryotic cells contain several different organelles. **Skill: Cell Structure, Function, and Type.**

38. C. Animals and plants are examples of eukaryotes. Because seaweed is a type of plant, it is a eukaryote. A virus is not a cell; it is neither prokaryotic nor eukaryotic. **Skill: Cell Structure, Function, and Type.**

39. D. The ATP provides the reducing power to make carbon dioxide into sugar. **Skill: Cellular Reproduction, Cellular Respiration, and Photosynthesis.**

40. B. Chlorophyll comes from chloroplasts, which are structures found in plant cells. Leaves contain chlorophyll, which is required for photosynthesis. **Skill: Cellular Reproduction, Cellular Respiration, and Photosynthesis.**

41. **A.** Mitosis and meiosis are both ways that cells divide to produce new cells. However, mitosis can produce new cells asexually by using one parent cell. Meiosis requires two parent cells to produce daughter cells. **Skill: Cellular Reproduction, Cellular Respiration, and Photosynthesis.**

42. **A.** Diploid refers to the full number of chromosomes. **Skill: Genetics and DNA.**

43. **C.** In a DNA molecule, cytosine can only pair with guanine. **Skill: Genetics and DNA.**

44. **C.** The placebo is a false treatment given to a group to account for the body's psychological response to this type of treatment in a study. **Skill: Designing an Experiment.**

45. **D.** The variable that is manipulated, or what is administered to a group as a treatment, is called the treatment group. **Skill: Designing an Experiment.**

46. **A.** During experimental analysis, results from data collection are analyzed for cause-and-effect relationships. **Skill: Designing an Experiment.**

47. **A.** Empirical evidence provides data and experimental setups that are repeatable by other people. **Skill: Designing an Experiment.**

48. **B.** Because iron-54 and iron-56 are isotopes of the same element, they have the same number of protons and the same atomic number, but the numbers of neutrons and mass numbers are different. **Skill: Scientific Notation.**

49. **A.** The atomic number for tin is 50, which means all atoms of tin have 50 protons. To determine the number of neutrons, subtract the number of protons from the mass number: 120 − 50 = 70 neutrons. Because the atom is neutral, it has 50 electrons to balance the charge of the protons. **Skill: Scientific Notation.**

50. **D.** There is one sodium atom in the reactants and two atoms of sodium in the products, so sodium is unbalanced. **Skill: Chemical Equations.**

51. **D.** In a polar molecule, one end of the molecule is slightly negative, and the other end is slightly positive. **Skill: Properties of Matter.**

52. **C.** Net water movement through a membrane in response to the concentration of a solute is called osmosis. **Skill: Properties of Matter.**

53. **D.** In a solid, particles have the least amount of energy and do not move as much as they do in other states of matter. The strong cohesive forces between the particles keep them close together. **Skill: States of Matter.**

Section IV. English and Language Usage

1. **A.** May. Months, days, and holidays need to be capitalized, and seasons do not need to be. **Skill: Capitalization.**

2. C. *I go to bed early so I do not feel tired.* There should be a comma before *so* as it is a coordinating conjunction. **Skill: Punctuation.**

3. B. *Business* is the only correct spelling. **Skill: Spelling.**

4. D. *Safely* is an adverb that describes the verb *traveled.* **Skill: Adjectives and Adverbs.**

5. B. *The* is an article, not a conjunction. **Skill: Conjunctions and Prepositions.**

6. B. To make the word *frog* plural, simply add *-s.* **Skill: Nouns.**

7. C. *Whom* is a pronoun. **Skill: Pronouns.**

8. C. The subject is *Mai and her friend Oksana,* and the predicate is *love to ride roller coasters.* **Skill: Subject and Verb Agreement.**

9. A. In a command like this one, the "understood" subject is *you.* **Skill: Subject and Verb Agreement.**

10. A. *Did* is a helping verb; *ask* is the main verb. **Skill: Verbs and Verb Tenses.**

11. D. *Unless.* The word *unless* signifies the beginning of a dependent clause and is the only conjunction that makes sense in the sentence. **Skill: Types of Clauses.**

12. C. *Which.* The word *which* signifies the beginning of a dependent clause and is the only conjunction that makes sense in the sentence. **Skill: Types of Clauses.**

13. B. *Yet.* It is the only conjunction that fits within the context of the sentence. **Skill: Types of Clauses.**

14. C. This is a compound sentence joining two independent clauses with a comma and the conjunction *but.* **Skill: Types of Sentences.**

15. A. This option would make the sentence a simple sentence. **Skill: Types of Sentences.**

16. D. I gotta go to school. It is the sentence that uses the most slang. **Skill: Formal and Informal Language.**

17. C. Congratulations on your recent success. It is the sentence with the most formal language and no slang. **Skill: Formal and Informal Language.**

18. C. It's sort of a bad time. The sentence has contractions and uses informal and slang words. **Skill: Formal and Informal Language.**

19. B. The meaning of <u>bolt</u> in the context of this sentence is "a quick movement in a particular direction." **Skill: Context Clues and Multiple Meaning Words.**

20. D. The meaning of <u>bind</u> in this context is "to form a mass that stays connected." The word "together" helps you figure out which meaning of <u>bind</u> is being used. **Skill: Context Clues and Multiple Meaning Words.**

21. C. The meaning of <u>emulate</u> in this context is "to try to be like someone you admire." The word "imitate" helps you figure out the meaning of <u>emulate</u>. **Skill: Context Clues and Multiple Meaning Words.**

22. D. The meaning of <u>novice</u> in the context of this sentence is "beginner." **Skill: Context Clues and Multiple Meaning Words.**

23. D. The word "leaves" has more than one meaning. **Skill: Context Clues and Multiple Meaning Words**

24. D. The suffix that means "in a manner of or resembling" is *-esque* as in the word *grotesque*. **Skill: Root Words, Prefixes, and Suffixes.**

25. C. The root that means "people" is *dem* as in the word *democracy*. **Skill: Root Words, Prefixes, and Suffixes.**

26. A. The prefix that means "former" is *ex-* as in the word *ex-husband*. **Skill: Root Words, Prefixes, and Suffixes.**

27. B. The prefix *mono-* means "one" so a monolingual person would only know how to speak one language. **Skill: Root Words, Prefixes, and Suffixes.**

28. B. The prefix *bi-* means "two," so *bilateral* means "relating to two sides." **Skill: Root Words, Prefixes, and Suffixes.**

TEAS PRACTICE EXAM 2

SECTION I. READING

You have 64 minutes to complete 53 questions.

Please read the text below and answer questions 1-3.

In the past 10-15 years, koalas have been repeatedly harmed or killed in traffic accidents. When the animals cross busy roads, highways, and intersections to get to their food source, the eucalyptus tree, many of them meet a terrible fate. Australian developers have been taking over koala habitats to keep up with the country's booming population. This has resulted in the endangerment of the country's most beloved animal. Concerned individuals have taken action by creating koala "pathways," routes traveling over roads, highways, and intersections to ensure koalas keep safe. In addition, koala hospitals have been established in these areas to rehabilitate the injured animals.

1. **Which phrase best describes the topic of the group of sentences above?**

   A. An analysis of animal behavior in the wild

   B. An account of human impact on an animal species

   C. A description of a building development plan

   D. An examination of the ways humans help animals

2. **Which of the following sentences would best function as a topic sentence to unite the text?**

   A. Over 4,000 koalas are hurt or injured each year by automobiles.

   B. Koalas spend most of their time in trees but need to occasionally travel across roads to move around.

   C. Human encroachment on natural habitats has negatively impacted the koala population.

   D. Australia's building development projects have tripled over the past decade.

3. **Which sentence provides another supporting detail to address the topic of the text?**

   A. Kangaroos, emus, and wombats are other popular animals in Australia.

   B. Australia has a diverse population of citizens from various countries throughout the world.

   C. Koalas are not bears but marsupials, mammals that carry their young in a pouch.

   D. Australia has erected over 500 koala pathways over the past two years.

Read the text below and answer questions 4-5.

Carving a pumpkin is a fun activity that can create family memories to last a lifetime.

You Will Need

A pumpkin
A knife or kid-safe cutting tool
A bowl
A large spoon
A marker
Old newspapers or plastic sheeting (optional)
Your imagination!

What to Do

Before you start carving a pumpkin, choose your workspace carefully. Spread newspapers or plastic sheeting over the floor if desired.

First, hollow the pumpkin out. Do this by using your knife or kid-safe cutting tool to make a circular cut on the pumpkin around the stem. Carefully pull off the outer rind and reach into the pumpkin to scoop out the pulp and seeds. Scrape the bottom and inside edges of the pumpkin with the spoon to remove as much pulp as possible. A jack-o-lantern with a wet, pulpy interior is difficult to carve and rots quickly once it is on display.

Now it is time to create your jack-o-lantern's face. Clean the surface of the pumpkin if necessary and decide which side you'll use for the face. Errors cannot easily be fixed once you start to carve, so for best results, draw the design onto the pumpkin before making any cuts. Then use your knife or cutting tool to carefully carve your jack-o-lantern's features.

4. **Which step comes just before the creation of the jack-o-lantern's face?**

   A. Scooping out the pulp

   B. Cutting around the stem

   C. Rotting while on display

   D. Preparing the workspace

5. **Why is it best to draw a design onto the pumpkin before cutting?**

   A. It prevents injury.

   B. It prevents errors.

   C. It prevents rotting.

   D. It prevents messes.

Read the following text and then answer questions 6-8.

Preheat your oven to 350 degrees. Get out all your equipment and ingredients. In a large bowl, combine flour, baking powder, sugar, and salt. Then soften 1 cup of butter. Next add the butter and the eggs to the dry mixture and stir until all the ingredients are mixed. Mix in the chocolate chips. Using a tablespoon, spoon out the batter onto a pre-greased cookie sheet. Bake in the oven for 12 minutes. Allow cookies to cool before serving.

6. **Which of the following words from the text indicate sequence?**

   A. Preheat, Mix   C. Using, Bake

   B. Then, Next   D. Get, In

7. **What does the term "pre-greased cookie sheet" tell you?**

    A. That you are supposed to grease the cookie sheet right after you spoon out the batter

    B. That you are supposed to grease the cookie sheet at some time before putting the batter onto it

    C. That you are supposed to grease the cookie sheet after preheating the oven

    D. That you are supposed to grease the cookie sheet after the baking the cookies

8. **What sequence word would best fit at the beginning of this sentence from the text?**

    Allow cookies to cool before serving.

    A. Then   C. After

    B. Last   D. Next

Read the following draft essay and answer questions 9-16.

As a child, I loved to chase butterflies in my grandmother's garden. (1) Now that I have children, I'm saddened there are so few butterflies left. Keeping butterfly populations healthy enriches lives and sustains ecosystems. (2) For this reason, I feel the Kingfield County Commission should support the effort to create habitat for butterflies and other pollinators along our highways. (3)

Kingfield's two major highways, Highway 65 and Highway 18, are both lined by grassy strips of unused land that the county maintains at taxpayer expense. (4) Currently, maintenance on these strips involves periodic mowing and pesticide spraying to keep back weeds.

(5) This practice harms butterflies and prevents the growth of plants that can sustain them. (6) To create pollinator habitat, we would need to change the way we manage our highways. (7) Instead of mowing and spraying, we could plant wildflowers such as white milkweed and transform the green strips into meadows that would support a wide variety of butterfly and other pollinator species. (8)

This project would cost surprisingly little. (9) State and federal organizations have grant programs in place to support set-up costs such as the purchase of wildflower seed for pollinator habitat creation. Long-term maintenance would demand only occasional maintenance to keep wildflowers away from roadways and reduce wildfire risk. Costs could be minimized by tapping local environmental and gardening groups for volunteer help. (10) "The members of our horticultural society are extremely generous with their time when it comes to promoting conservation efforts." (11)

Some gardeners might balk at the idea of intentionally planting milkweed and other wildflowers that are sometimes considered undesirable. It is true that wildflowers spread into fields and gardens whose owners do not want them. But those gardens need butterflies and other pollinators to remain healthy.

A low-cost effort to save butterflies could enrich our lives for many years to come and make gardens healthier. (12) With a little effort, we can make sure there are butterflies for our grandchildren to chase someday. (13)

9. Which sentence is the thesis statement?

   A. Sentence 1   C. Sentence 3

   B. Sentence 2   D. Sentence 6

10. In this draft, the flow of ideas from the introduction to the first body paragraph is a little unclear. Which sentence, if it appeared at the beginning of the first body paragraph, would make a clearer link back to the thesis?

    A. Sentence 5   C. Sentence 7

    B. Sentence 6   D. Sentence 8

11. Which revision of sentence 9 links more clearly back to the main idea?

    A. This type of pollinator habitat creation costs surprisingly little.

    B. Some might object that this project would cost surprisingly little.

    C. The cost of this project would come in county jobs, not money.

    D. The low cost of this project could create an opportunity to lower taxes.

12. Which evidence would strengthen the argument outlined in Sentence 9?

    A. Statistics showing a 35-year decline in the monarch butterfly population

    B. Scientific evidence connecting pesticide use to butterfly population decline

    C. A breakdown of the costs of a similar project completed in a nearby county

    D. Surveys of schoolchildren showing that most of them love to chase butterflies

13. What should the writer do to improve sentence 11?

    A. Identify the speaker

    B. Restate the idea in different words

    C. Define *horticultural*

    D. Place the sentence elsewhere

14. Reread the third body paragraph:

    Some gardeners might balk at the idea of intentionally planting milkweed and other wildflowers that are sometimes considered undesirable. It is true that wildflowers spread into fields and gardens whose owners do not want them. But those gardens need butterflies and other pollinators to remain healthy.

    What should the writer do to strengthen this paragraph?

    A. Outline beneficial properties of milkweed and other wildflowers, such as medicinal uses

    B. Offer evidence to support the point that butterflies and other pollinators keep gardens healthy

    C. Claim that wildflowers will not spread from highway habitat strips into local fields and gardens

    D. Eliminate the suggestion that some people might not like the idea of creating pollinator habitat

15. **Which sentence most clearly improves sentence 12 in the context of the essay?**

    A. By creating habitat on public land near highways, it can save the butterflies and other pollinators that enrich our lives and keep our gardens healthy.

    B. By creating habitat on public land near highways, we can save the butterflies and other pollinators that enrich our lives and keep our gardens healthy.

    C. Saving the butterflies and other pollinators that enrich our lives and keep our gardens healthy is the right thing to do because otherwise they will go extinct.

    D. Saving the butterflies and other pollinators that enrich our lives and keep our gardens healthy is the right thing to do because extinction is the clear alternative.

16. **Which type of ending would likely be a more effective ending than sentence 13?**

    A. A quotation from a textbook describing the anatomical parts of a monarch butterfly

    B. An implicit suggestion that it would be selfish deny support to the pollinator habitat proposal

    C. A request that the reader take a specific action to support the proposal to create pollinator habitat

    D. A reference to a study suggesting that many species on Earth may soon die out if we do not take action

Read the draft paragraph below and answer questions 17-21.

The Harry Potter books are told from a third person limited omniscient point of view. (1) The narrator describes Harry's actions using words like *he* and *him* rather than *I* and *me*, but the narrator can access Harry's inner thoughts as a real human observer could not. (2) The narrator is unable to read the thoughts of other characters, even of Harry's close friends, Ron and Hermione. (3) The reader must guess at their thoughts, as friends must sometimes guess at the thoughts of friends in real life. (4) Rowling weaves her narratives in a way that makes readers feel a close kinship with Harry. (5)

17. **Imagine this is a body paragraph in a draft essay with the following thesis:**

    "The *Harry Potter* series is successful partly because the author, J.K. Rowling, does an expert job of engaging her audience's emotions."

    Which sentence should be moved to the beginning of the paragraph to create a clear and direct link back to this argument?

    A. Sentence 2   C. Sentence 4

    B. Sentence 3   D. Sentence 5

18. Which evidence would back up the claim that the Harry Potter books are told in the third person limited omniscient point of view?

   A. A detail describing emotional events in the life of author J.K. Rowling

   B. A quotation that shows Harry feeling surprised by another character's choices

   C. An example of how the author's word choice makes the setting scene magical

   D. A short summary of an exciting scene in which a character encounters a dragon

19. Which transition *best* fits at the beginning of Sentence 2?

   A. That is

   C. In contrast

   B. Moreover

   D. Thereafter

20. Which transition *best* fits at the beginning of Sentence 4?

   A. Therefore

   C. Seemingly

   B. In contrast

   D. Meanwhile

21. Which sentence provides further explanation to back up the point in Sentence 4?

   A. This fact is surprising since the characters are supposed to be magical, so they should be able to read each other's minds.

   B. When readers share a character's knowledge and perspective in this way, they are more likely to connect emotionally with his story.

   C. You have probably had the real-life experience of wondering what friends were thinking and feeling worried about their opinions.

   D. Readers must wonder whether author J.K. Rowling feels socially anxious when she is unable to read her friends' thoughts.

Read the passage below and answer questions 22-28.

When my 13-year-old daughter entered the house, the door slammed open with a celebratory "bang!" I was instantly dismayed to see that my first-born stomped right by me as I held my arms open for a warm hug.

"How was your day, honey?" I asked as she gave me her quintessential eye roll.

I sat across from her ready to hear how marvelous her day was. However, I only got an earful of all the drama that had ensued at school: "So-and-so said this," "gym was a drag," "Mr. Fletcher doesn't like me because I am not a math genius."

My head ached from nodding so much, so I got up quickly to bring her something.

"Mom! How could you get up when I'm in the middle of telling you about my life?" she barked.

Despite her protest, her eyes could not help but light up when I brought her a freshly baked chocolate chip cookie on a plate.

I guess life isn't all that bad, is it?

22. **Which adjectives best describe the tone of the passage?**

    A. Ironic, furious

    B. Honest, furious

    C. Ironic, amusing

    D. Honest, amusing

23. **Which sentence from the passage is clearly ironic?**

    A. "How was your day, honey?"

    B. I sat across from her ready to hear how marvelous her day was.

    C. My head ached from nodding so much, so I got up quickly to bring her something.

    D. "Mom! How could you get up when I'm in the middle of telling you about my life?"

24. **The author of the passage first establishes the ironic tone by:**

    A. describing the slamming of the door as "celebratory."

    B. quoting the daughter's words.

    C. explaining how the mother got up to get the daughter cookie.

    D. having the mother state that life "isn't all that bad."

25. **Reread the following sentence:**

    I guess life isn't all that bad, is it?

    Which adjective could describe an effective reader's mood when reading this line in the context of the passage?

    A. Entertained

    B. Frustrated

    C. Empathetic

    D. Dismissive

26. **Which word or phrase does *not* function as a transition in the passage?**

    A. Instantly   C. So

    B. However   D. Despite

27. **The transitions "however" and "despite" link ideas in the passage by showing:**

    A. when events happen in time.

    B. how certain ideas contrast.

    C. examples that illustrate ideas.

    D. cause-and-effect relationships.

28. **Reread the following sentence:**

    "How was your day, honey?" I asked as she gave me her quintessential eye roll.

    Which transition would you use if the next sentence describes the daughter *also* making a "tsk" sound to show her frustration?

    A. Finally   C. To illustrate

    B. Furthermore   D. Nevertheless

29. **Read the sentences below.**

    There are so many entries for the County Chili Cookoff, it is going to be a challenge to choose just one winner. It's also going to be a pleasure to taste them.

    Which word functions as a transition?

    A. There   C. Also

    B. One   D. Going

Read the passages below and answer questions 30-33.

Many people find termites to be destructive little pests, but they are actually ingenious little creatures. If you were to look at a termite mound, you would see first hand how incredible these insects are.

These masters of construction work together to erect high-functioning, green-energy skyscrapers out of nothing but soil, saliva, and dung. The largest one documented is in the Democratic Republic of the Congo. This mound, measuring 12.8 meters (41.9 feet) tall, has heat regulation and air conditioning systems. It also contains numerous chambers for food storage, gardens, and babies.

And just think: a termite is only .6 cm long, yet it is still capable of building a sophisticated structure that's 2,013 times its size!

*

As we hiked along the dusty trail deep within the Congo, our tour guide suddenly stopped and held up his hand.

Panic rose inside me, as I expected to see a ghastly hyena or other vicious predator in our midst. But he slowly pointed toward a large mound off the side of the path.

What on earth?

It rose high above us, a tall, sandy structure, its arms outstretched to the sky.

"This," he began in a whisper so as not to disturb its inhabitants, "is a termite mound. Inside are thousands of termites.

These tiny little insects have worked together to build this massive structure. And not only is it ventilated to keep them cool, but there are tons of little rooms or chambers inside for different purposes."

WHOA. A termite mound? How on earth did those pesky little bugs do that?

30. **What is the purpose of the first paragraph of Passage 1?**
    A. To inform   C. To persuade
    B. To distract   D. To entertain

31. **What is the primary purpose of Passage 2?**
    A. To inform   C. To persuade
    B. To distract   D. To entertain

32. **With which statement would the author of Passage 1 most likely agree with?**
    A. Things are not always what they seem.
    B. The best things in life come in small packages.
    C. If you try hard enough, you can achieve anything.
    D. Working together accomplishes more than working alone.

33. **The author of Passage 1 supports his/her points primarily by:**
    A. telling humanizing stories.
    B. relying on facts and logic.
    C. pointing to expert sources.
    D. using fear tactics and manipulation.

34. **Which phrase describes the set of techniques an author uses to support an argument or develop a main idea?**

    A. Points of view

    B. Logical fallacies

    C. Statistical analyses

    D. Rhetorical strategies

35. **An author's point of view is a(n):**

    A. lack of purpose.

    B. general outlook.

    C. rhetorical strategy.

    D. appeal to the emotions.

36. **The author's _____ is the reason for writing.**

    A. purpose

    B. rhetoric

    C. main idea

    D. point of view

Read the passages below and answer questions 37-40.

As a parent, I find television and movie rating systems unhelpful. Ratings systems are not human. Their scores are based on numbers: how many bad words, how many gory scenes. To me, that makes no sense. Nobody else knows my kids like I do, so nobody else can say what's okay for them to watch.

In my experience, the content a government organization rates as PG or PG-13 may or may not be appropriate for my 9-, 14-, and 16-year-olds. My youngest is quite mature for his age, and I'm fine with him hearing a bad word or two as a part of a meaningful story.

Violence concerns me more. I won't let even my 16-year-old watch frivolous violence or horror. But I don't shelter him from realistic violence. My little guy still

has to stay out of the room for the bloody stuff. But eventually, kids need to know what's out there.

37. **The primary purpose of this passage is to:**

    A. decide.

    B. inform.

    C. persuade.

    D. entertain.

38. **The author of this passage would be most likely to agree that:**

    A. kids should not watch television or movies at all until they are in their teens.

    B. government rating systems should have more levels to make them more useful.

    C. it is never appropriate to prevent any human being from watching any show or movie.

    D. another parent should have the right to let her own kids watch extremely violent movies.

39. **The author of this passage would be likely to support an effort to:**

    A. create a government system to recommend ages for reading children's books.

    B. prevent kids from attending movies in the theater without their parents' presence.

    C. provide parents more information about the content of children's shows and movies.

    D. change the age for watching PG-13 movies down to 10 because today's kids are more savvy.

40. What is the most likely reason for the author's decision to include the phrase "as a parent" at the beginning?

    A. This phrase provides a reason to support her opinion.

    B. She is implying that non-parents cannot know what kids need.

    C. This phrase provides a transition from the points she made earlier.

    D. She is establishing herself as a knowledgeable source on this topic.

41. What is a text feature?

    A. A movie adaptation of a book

    B. An unwritten summary of a text

    C. A group of contiguous paragraphs

    D. An element that stands out from a text

Read the following passage and answer questions 42-46.

Most children under the age of 18 are very overweight. Statistics show that 1 in 3 children have been diagnosed as obese. This is way too much. There is no reason for so many children to be obese. Children must eat a balanced diet devoid of processed foods, get at least one hour of exercise every day, and make sure to sleep for 9-10 hours or suffer a life full of health problems. It is concerning to see so many unhealthy young people in our country. Children should be active and engaged instead of sedentary and apathetic.

42. What is the primary argument in the passage?

    A. A healthy diet is the key to a healthy life.

    B. Childhood obesity is a major problem in our country.

    C. Too many young people do not get enough sleep each night.

    D. Processed foods have caused too much obesity in our youth.

43. Which excerpt from the text, if true, is a fact?

    A. Most children under the age of 18 are very overweight.

    B. Statistics show that 1 in 3 children have been diagnosed as obese.

    C. It is concerning to see so many unhealthy young people in our country.

    D. Children should be active and engaged instead of sedentary and apathetic.

44. Re-read the following sentence from the passage:

Children must eat a balanced diet devoid of processed foods, get at least one hour of exercise every day, and make sure to sleep for 9-10 hours or suffer a life full of health problems.

What type of faulty reasoning does this sentence display?

    A. Either/or fallacy

    B. Circular reasoning

    C. Bandwagon argument

    D. False statement of cause and effect

45. Re-read the following sentence from the passage:

There is no reason for so many children to be obese.

The reasoning in this sentence is faulty because it:

A. suggests that this is an issue that needs attention.

B. claims that there are many ways to solve this problem.

C. restates the argument in different words instead of providing evidence.

D. assumes that children are overweight based on their own choices.

46. Re-read the following sentence from the passage:

Most children under the age of 18 are very overweight.

This sentence is an opinion because it:

A. reflects a belief, not a verifiable fact.

B. does not say how much "very" is.

C. restricts its statement to children under 18.

D. lumps all people under 18 into one category.

47. A statement that is probably true is a(n):

A. fact.

B. claim.

C. opinion.

D. argument.

48. **Which of the following is an example of a primary source?**

A. An encyclopedia

B. A biography

C. A guidebook

D. An interview

Read the following passage and answer questions 49-52.

You know what I hate? Businesses that rely on contract workers and freelancers instead of regular employees.

Don't hit me with arguments about grater freedom for workers. Freedom isn't free if your bleeding out in the street.

Sound the alarm, people! Workers are suffering! No benefits means you're out of luck if you get sick and can't do your job. Plus, studies show freelancers don't make as much money as regular employees.

--From Rod's Job Blog at rodtalksaboutjobs.com

49. **Which of the following is not a sign that the reader should be skeptical of this source?**

A. The passage contains typos and spelling errors.

B. The author presents opinion information as if it is fact.

C. There is no clear information about the author's credentials.

D. The passage comes from a personal blog with a .com address.

50. **Why should a reader be skeptical of the point about freelancers not making as much money as regular employees?**

A. The argument is not based in logic.

B. Some freelancers make plenty of money.

C. The source of the information is not clear.

D. The sentence contains grammatical errors.

51. **A reader should be skeptical of the line "Freedom isn't free if your (sic) bleeding out in the street" because it:**

    A. appears to use objective language but is actually hiding gender bias.

    B. uses emotional language without responding to the opposing argument.

    C. seems to present an expert point of view but does not name the source.

    D. makes no attempt to defend regular workers in a discussion of the economy.

52. **A student is writing a paper on employment trends and wants to quote an expert's opinion. What type of site would provide the most credible alternative to Rod's Job Blog?**

    A. A different post on Rod's Jobs Blog

    B. A different blog with a .net address

    C. An opinion article by a recognized expert in the field

    D. A government website tracking employment statistics

53. **The theme of a text is:**

    A. nonfiction but not narrative.

    B. narrative but not nonfiction.

    C. suggested but not stated outright.

    D. stated outright, not just suggested.

SECTION II. MATHEMATICS

You have 54 minutes to complete 36 questions.

1. The bar chart shows the number of boys and girls who participate in sports. What year had the most participants?

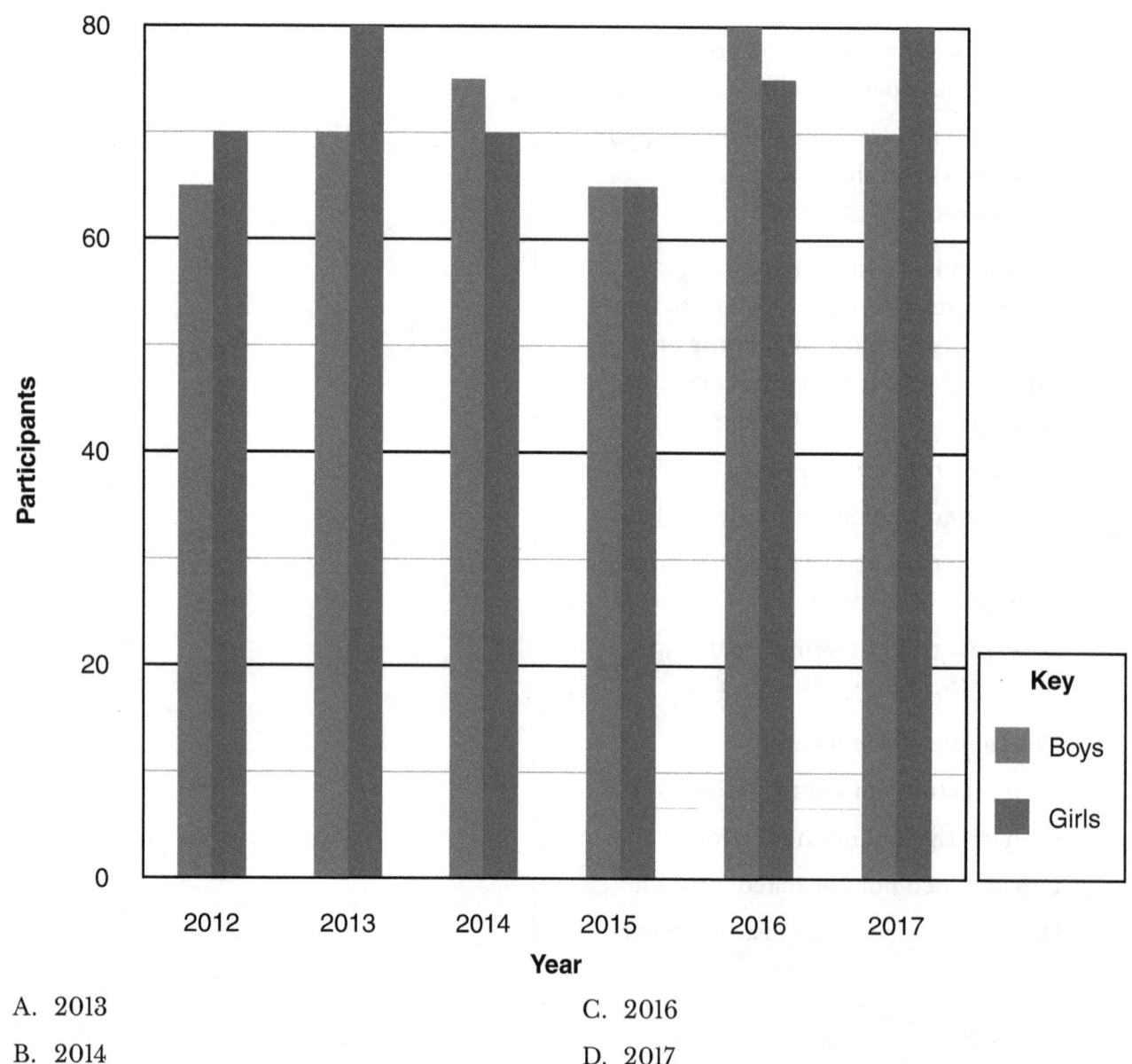

Sports Participants

A. 2013

B. 2014

C. 2016

D. 2017

2. If a customer wants to give her waiter a 22% tip on her $37 bill, how much will her total bill cost?

   A. $57.35   C. $48.68

   B. $38.68   D. $45.14

3. Two siblings each took a standardized math test for their grade levels. One sibling took the test with 75 questions and the older sibling took the test with 140 questions. If the younger sibling got 60 questions right and both siblings received the same overall score, how many questions did the older sibling answer correctly?

   A. 125   C. 112

   B. 105   D. 122

4. Change 0.375 to a fraction. Simplify completely.

   A. $\frac{3}{8}$ C. $\frac{1}{2}$

   B. $\frac{2}{5}$ D. $\frac{7}{16}$

5. The level of a river during a flood was 39.45 feet. After a week, the water level declined to 18.97 feet. What was the amount of decrease in feet?

   A. 20.38   C. 21.38

   B. 20.48   D. 21.48

6. A woman deposits $4,200 into a savings account that earns 3.25% annual interest. If she never adds any more money to the account, how much money will she have in a year?

   A. $5,336.00   C. $5,536.50

   B. $4,336.50   D. $4,136.00

7. $\frac{1}{8} + \frac{4}{5}$

   A. $\frac{37}{40}$ C. $\frac{5}{13}$

   B. $\frac{7}{8}$ D. $\frac{5}{8}$

8. What is 15% of 64?

   A. 5:48   C. 48:5

   B. 15:64   D. 64:15

9. A small landscaping company mows lawns and has three 5.4-gallon gas cans. One day, the landscapers empty the gas cans three times. How many gallons of gas did they use?

   A. 10.8   C. 32.4

   B. 16.2   D. 48.6

10. A mom gets off of work late and needs to pick up her child from daycare immediately. She has to drive 18 miles in 20 minutes. On average, how fast does she need to drive?

    A. 45 mph   C. 54 mph

    B. 60 mph   D. 62 mph

11. $1\frac{1}{2} + \frac{2}{3}$

    A. $\frac{5}{6}$ C. $1\frac{5}{6}$

    B. $2\frac{1}{6}$ D. $1\frac{2}{5}$

12. A sponsored sports event wants to take any money from participant fees and give it to volunteers evenly. If the event costs $75 per participant and there are 320 participants, how much money can the event hope to give to each of its 12 volunteers?

    A. $3,840   C. $2,400

    B. $512   D. $2,000

13. The box plot shows the number of weekly sales by a business during the year. Which statement is true for the box plot?

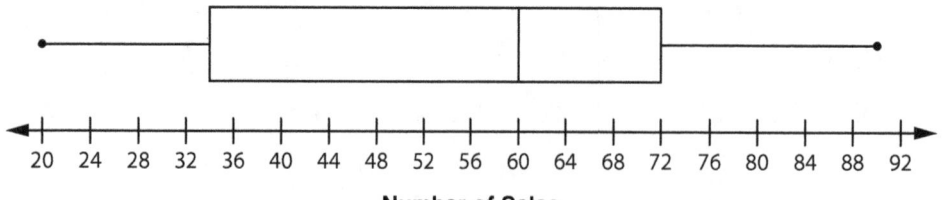

Number of Sales

A. The median is 34 sales.

B. The median is 72 sales.

C. The difference between the maximum and minimum is 40 sales.

D. The difference between the maximum and minimum is 70 sales.

14. Solve for the value of y when $x = 6$.

$y = (x^2 - 4) \div 8$

A. 3

B. 1

C. 4

D. 2

15. Perform the operation.

$(3y^3 - 4y^2 + 6y + 3) - (2y^3 - 3y)$

A. $5y^3 - 4y^2 + 3y + 3$

B. $y^3 - 4y^2 + 3y + 3$

C. $5y^3 - 4y^2 + 9y + 3$

D. $y^3 - 4y^2 + 9y + 3$

16. If a taxi costs $8.00 plus $3.85 per mile ($m$) and a customer needs to travel 14 miles, select the equation that represents how much the cab fare will cost.

A. $3.85m + $8.00 = $61.90

B. $8.00 \div m + $3.85 = $61.90

C. ($8.00 + 3.85)m = $61.90

D. $8.00m + $3.85 = $61.90

17. Convert 0.75 kilograms to grams. (Note: 1 kilogram is equal to 1,000 grams.)

A. 0.0075 grams

B. 0.075 grams

C. 75 grams

D. 750 grams

18. $2\frac{9}{10} \div 3\frac{1}{2}$

A. $\frac{2}{7}$

B. $\frac{9}{20}$

C. $\frac{2}{3}$

D. $\frac{29}{35}$

19. A student took a final exam with 175 questions. If the student got 50 questions wrong, approximately what percentage score did they earn?

A. 78%

B. 86%

C. 93%

D. 71%

20. Change 2.5 to a fraction. Simplify completely.

A. $2\frac{1}{8}$

B. $2\frac{1}{4}$

C. $2\frac{1}{3}$

D. $2\frac{1}{2}$

21. Samantha ran 8 kilometers in 50 minutes. If she ran that same pace, approximately how long will it take her to run 10 kilometers?

A. 86 minutes

B. 63 minutes

C. 90 minutes

D. 72 minutes

22. A half circle has an area of 45 square centimeters. Find the diameter to the nearest tenth of a centimeter. Use 3.14 for π.

    A. 2.7   C. 10.8

    B. 5.4   D. 16.2

23. Convert 9 meters to yards. (Note: 1 meter is equal to 1.093 yards.)

    A. 4.09 yards   C. 9.84 yards

    B. 8.23 yards   D. 12.28 yards

24. Karida has a part-time job. She works 4.25 hours on Thursday and Friday and 6.5 hours on Saturday and Sunday. What is her hourly rate if her check is $268.75?

    A. $8.50   C. $14.50

    B. $12.50   D. $21.50

25. Given the coordinates for a square $(-6,6), (6,6), (6,-6), (-6,-6)$, find the length of each side of the square.

    A. 0 units   C. 12 units

    B. 6 units   D. 18 units

26. Convert 72 pounds to kilograms. (Note: 1 pound is equal to 2.2 kilograms.)

    A. 32.73 kilograms   C. 144.0 kilograms

    B. 74.20 kilograms   D. 158.4 kilograms

27. A cube has a surface area of 54 square feet. What is the side length in feet? (Note: $SA = 6s^2$.)

    A. 2   C. 4

    B. 3   D. 5

28. Logan gets his hourly salary raised from $9.50 an hour to $10.25 an hour. What percentage did his wage increase?

    A. 9.3%   C. 7.5%

    B. 12.7%   D. 7.9%

29. Solve the equation for the unknown.

    $6x - 12 = -24$

    A. −4   C. 2

    B. −2   D. 4

30. $1\frac{9}{14} \div \frac{3}{5}$

    A. $\frac{69}{70}$ C. $1\frac{27}{70}$

    B. $1\frac{1}{3}$ D. $2\frac{31}{42}$

31. Write $0.\overline{1}$ as a percent.

    A. $0.\overline{1}\%$ C. $11.\overline{1}\%$

    B. $1.\overline{1}\%$ D. $111.\overline{1}\%$

32. If 1 out of every 250 people will contract a certain disease, what percent of people will contract it?

    A. 0.004%   C. 2.5%

    B. 0.4%   D. 25%

33. Solve for x when $(2^2)x = 5^2 - 1$.

    A. 4   C. 6

    B. 10   D. 8

34. Solve the equation for the unknown.

    $3x + 8 = 12$

    A. $\frac{3}{4}$ C. $\frac{4}{3}$

    B. 1   D. 2

35. The line chart shows the number of cars sold each month. Which month shows the greatest gain?

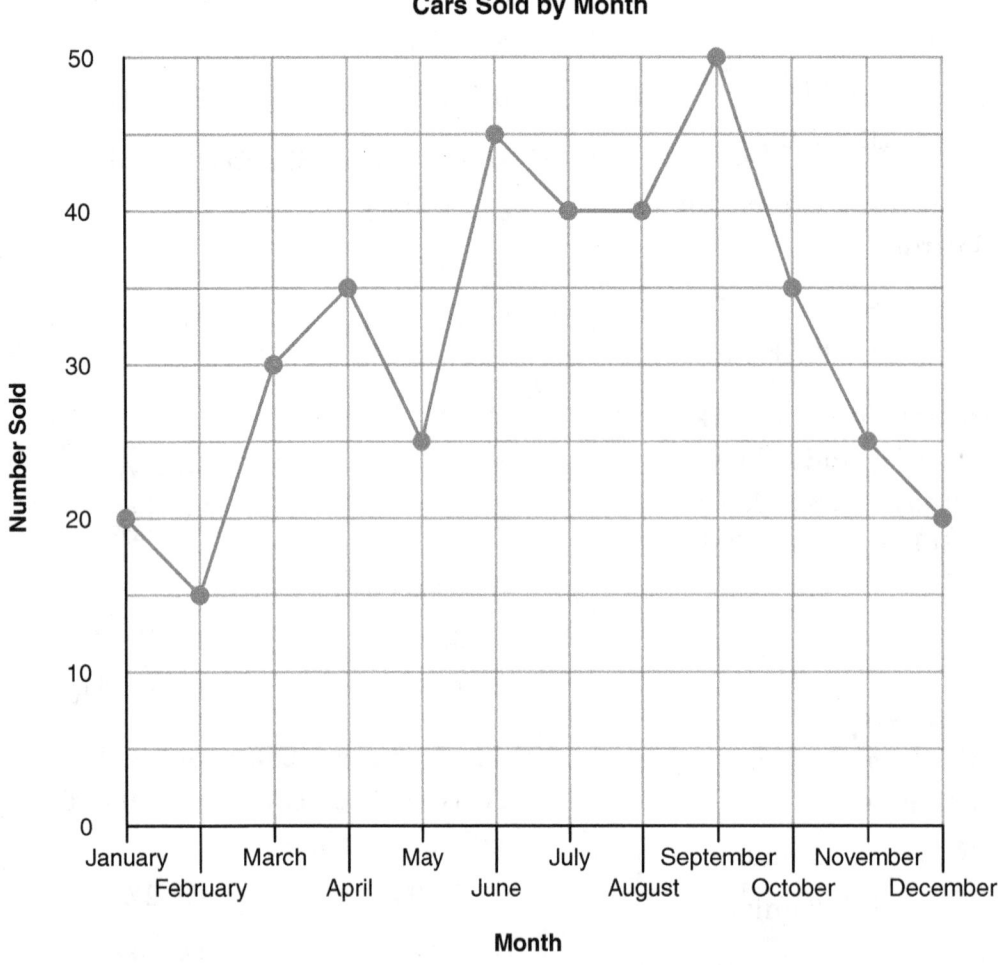

Cars Sold by Month

A. February to March

B. March to April

C. May to June

D. August to September

36. The dot plot shows the results of a favorite pet survey given to children. Each dot represents 5 respondents. Which statement is true for the dot plot?

Favorite Pet

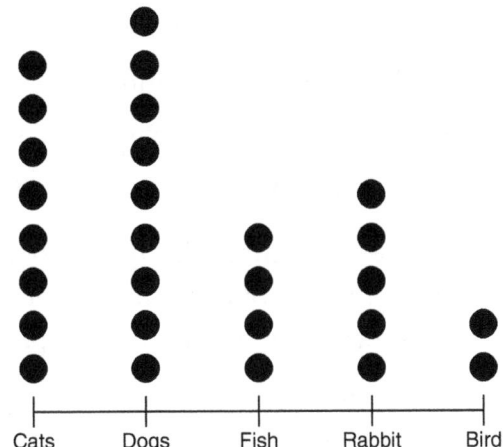

A. Fish was the favorite of four children.

B. There are 80 children who like cats or dogs.

C. There were 100 children asked about their favorite pet.

D. Less than half of the children like fish, rabbits, or birds.

SECTION III. SCIENCE

You have 63 minutes to complete 53 questions.

1. Which term represents a division of an organ from top to bottom?

   A. Coronal   C. Sagittal

   B. Midsagittal   D. Transverse

2. How many cavities make up the ventral cavity?

   A. Two   C. Five

   B. Three   D. Nine

3. After blood leaves the aorta, it travels to the

   A. arteries.   C. capillaries.

   B. arterioles.   D. venules.

4. Which formed element is found in the buffy coat?

   A. Epithelial cells

   B. Red blood cells

   C. White blood cells

   D. Endothelium cells

5. Which of the following hormones usually remains unchanged as a person ages?

   A. Adrenocorticotropic

   B. Epinephrine

   C. Prolactin

   D. Thyroid

6. Which two hormones promote sperm cell production in males?

   A. Growth and thyroid-stimulating

   B. Follicle-stimulating and prolactin

   C. Luteinizing and follicle-stimulating

   D. Thyroid-stimulating and luteinizing

7. How does the human body ensure that a hormone does not influence other cells by connecting to the wrong receptor?

   A. Each hormone only fits its receptor.

   B. Receptors mark the hormone for connection.

   C. Immune cells guard receptor cells to inhibit the wrong connection.

   D. Hormones are attracted to the correct receptor because of polarity.

8. Which enzyme breaks down lipids?

   A. Amylase   C. Peptidase

   B. Lipase   D. Sucrase

9. Which of the following organs maintains a healthy pH level when a person eats an orange?

   A. Gallbladder   C. Pancreas

   B. Liver   D. Tongue

10. Which of the following enzymes breaks down proteins?

    A. Amylase

    B. Lactase

    C. Pepsin

    D. Sucrase

11. **What is a source of UV radiation?**

    A. Tanning bed

    B. Indoor lighting

    C. Topical products

    D. Outdoor irritants

12. **Which describes the primary function of hair?**

    A. Protect the surface of the skin

    B. Prevent heat loss from the head

    C. Fight off various microbial infections

    D. Excrete toxic substances from the body

13. **Where are epidermal cells found before traveling to the skin's surface?**

    A. Stratum basale

    B. Stratum lucidum

    C. Stratum corneum

    D. Stratum granulosum

14. **Which of the following organs was never considered vestigial?**

    A. Adenoids   C. Spleen

    B. Appendix   D. Tonsils

15. **Which of the following results in allergies?**

    A. Histamines building up in the sinuses

    B. The immune system reacting to pollen

    C. The immune system overreacting to a particular substance

    D. The body's immune system breaking down

16. **Which gland is only active from birth through puberty?**

    A. Adenoids   C. Thymus

    B. Appendix   D. Tonsils

17. **Which of the following do B cells label invaders to be destroyed by:**

    A. Antibodies   C. Proteins

    B. Macrophages   D. T cells

18. **Which structure cushions bones at the point where they meet?**

    A. Joint   C. Ligament

    B. Tendon   D. Sarcomere

19. **Which of the following is a characteristic of all muscle types?**

    A. Striated in appearance

    B. Under voluntary control

    C. Shortens during contraction

    D. Stimulated by the nervous system

20. **What is the cytoplasm of the skeletal muscle fiber referred to as?**

    A. Myofibril   C. Sarcolemma

    B. Perimysium   D. Sarcoplasm

21. **What part of the nervous system controls blood vessel contraction?**

    A. Autonomic   C. Somatic

    B. Central   D. Sympathetic

22. **Where is genetic information found in a neuron?**

    A. Axon   C. Cell body

    B. Dendrite   D. Axon terminal

23. **What sense bypasses the thalamus as the CNS processes sensory information?**

    A. Hearing   C. Smelling

    B. Seeing   D. Touching

24. The basic human body plan, with the fundamental structures, organs, and systems, is developed at the end of which period?

    A. Embryogenesis

    B. Fertilization

    C. Gestation

    D. Puberty

25. The ova are analogous to which component of the male reproductive system?

    A. Foreskin   C. Sperm

    B. Scrotum   D. Testis

26. What happens as the diaphragm relaxes?

    A. The rib cage moves outward.

    B. Oxygen is brought into the lungs.

    C. Surface area of the alveoli increases.

    D. Carbon dioxide is removed from the body.

27. The diaphragm is found

    A. next to the   C. at the base of
       heart.   the lungs.

    B. behind the   D. connected to
       nasal cavity.   the bronchi.

28. Which structure is part of the appendicular skeleton?

    A. Ribs   C. Pelvic girdle

    B. Skull   D. Vertebral
                              column

29. What is the function of flat bone?

    A. Plays a role in body posture

    B. Provides mechanical strength

    C. Increases rigidity in movement

    D. Serves as a site of muscle attachment

30. How many types of bone exist in the human body?

    A. 2   C. 7

    B. 5   D. 10

31. Roughly how many liters of blood flow through the kidneys each day?

    A. 75   C. 180

    B. 100   D. 425

32. After being produced by the kidneys, where does urine flow next?

    A. Ureter

    B. Urethra

    C. Renel vein

    D. Renal artery

33. How many hydrogen atoms are bonded to oxygen in water?

    A. 1   C. 3

    B. 2   D. 4

34. Fats and steroids belong to what biomolecule class?

    A. Lipids   C. Nucleic acids

    B. Proteins   D. Carbohydrates

35. Where does enzyme synthesis occur in a cell?

    A. Cytoplasm

    B. Mitochondrion

    C. Nucleus

    D. Ribosome

36. Which organelle is associated with an animal cell?

    A. Cell wall   C. Chloroplast

    B. Flagellum   D. Golgi
                         apparatus

37. **Before mitosis occurs**

    A. the spindle fibers must elongate.

    B. DNA must wrap around histones.

    C. chromosomes must split into chromatids.

    D. the cell cycle process must be suspended.

38. **What molecule plays a direct role in chemiosmosis?**

    A. Glucose   C. O_2

    B. NADH   D. Pyruvate

39. **What is made only during the light reaction phase of photosynthesis?**

    A. ATP   C. H_2O

    B. CO_2 D. $FADH_2$

40. **What are the three parts of a nucleotide?**

    A. Sulfate group, five-carbon sugar molecule, and nitrogen base

    B. Phosphate group, five-carbon sugar molecule, and oxygen base

    C. Nitrogen base, phosphate group, and six-carbon sugar molecule

    D. Five-carbon sugar molecule, phosphate group, and nitrogen base

41. **What is the end product of translation?**

    A. Amino acids   C. Transfer RNA

    B. Stop codons   D. Messenger RNA

42. **The process that "rewrites" the information in a gene in DNA into a molecule of messenger RNA is called _____.**

    A. replication   C. transcription

    B. termination   D. translation

43. **How can an organism have two alleles for each trait but only one of those alleles is expressed?**

    A. One of the alleles is hidden in the chromosome.

    B. One of the alleles is dominant over the other allele.

    C. It depends on which allele is obtained from a parent first.

    D. The allele closest to the top of the chromosomes is expressed.

44. **What step of the scientific method relies on logic reasoning to be formulated?**

    A. Asking a question

    B. Writing a conclusion

    C. Researching information

    D. Developing a hypothesis

45. **A researcher wants to evaluate how different tire treads affect braking speed. How should she define her control group?**

    A. Number of tire treads tested

    B. Change in environmental conditions

    C. Braking distance measured over time

    D. Use of one car during the experiment

46. A study evaluated the impact of climate change on bird migration over time. The distance the birds traveled was measured for several years. What do the results show?

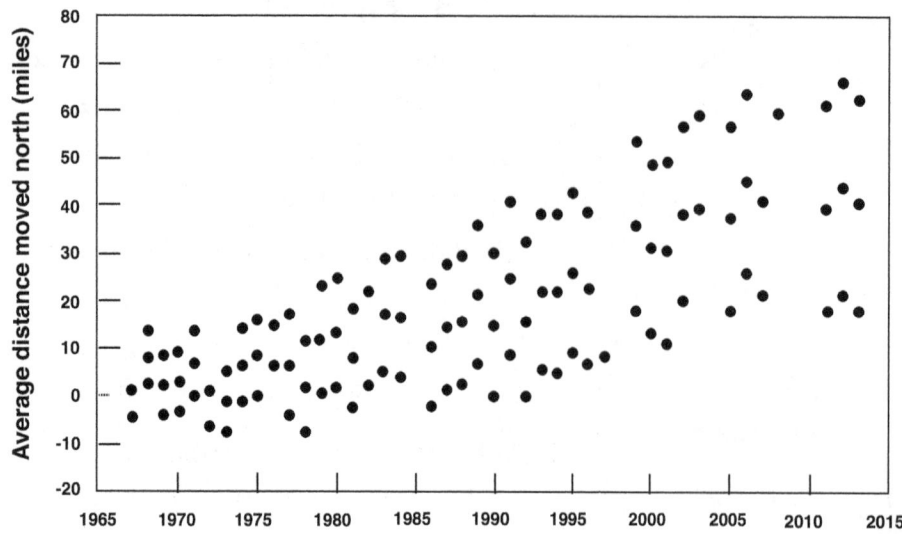

A. Bird migration increases over time.

B. Average distance is the highest in the 1970s.

C. There is a negative trend between migration and time.

D. Birds migrate at varying distances regardless of the year.

47. Which of the following atoms will have an overall negative charge?

A. 9 protons, 10 neutrons, 9 electrons

B. 12 protons, 13 neutrons, 10 electrons

C. 14 protons, 14 neutrons, 10 electrons

D. 15 protons, 16 neutrons, 18 electrons

48. Which of the following pairs of elements contains two elements in the same period?

A. Argon and neon

B. Zinc and cadmium

C. Beryllium and aluminum

D. Magnesium and aluminum

49. How many neutrons does an atom of silver-109 contain?

A. 47   C. 62

B. 60   D. 109

50. Why does oxygen diffuse out of lungs into the bloodstream?

A. The oxygen is repulsed by the blood.

B. The oxygen is being pulled into the blood.

C. The oxygen is polar, and the blood has the opposite charge.

D. The oxygen is going from a higher area of concentration to a lower one.

51. A student has attempted to balance the equation for the single-replacement reaction shown below, but it is still unbalanced. Which statement best describes how this equation is still unbalanced?

$$Mg + 2HCl \rightarrow MgCl_2 + 2H_2$$

A. There are more chlorine atoms in the reactants.

B. There are more chlorine atoms in the products.

C. There are more hydrogen atoms in the reactants.

D. There are more hydrogen atoms in the products.

52. What is the goal of diffusion?

A. Molecules traveling as far as they can

B. Molecules reaching equilibrium in an area

C. All molecules spreading to a different area

D. Molecules clustering around the densest area

53. When iron is exposed to water and oxygen, it corrodes. Why is this an example of a chemical property?

A. The iron gets weaker.

B. The iron changes color.

C. Rust is dangerous to the environment.

D. A new substance called iron (III) oxide (rust) is formed.

SECTION IV. ENGLISH AND LANGUAGE USAGE

You have 28 minutes to complete 28 questions.

1. **Which of the following is correct?**

   A. *Gone With The Wind*

   B. *Gone With the Wind*

   C. *Gone with the Wind*

   D. *Gone with the wind*

2. **What is the sentence with the correct use of punctuation?**

   A. Offcampus apartments are nicer.

   B. Off campus apartments are nicer.

   C. Off-campus apartments are nicer.

   D. Off-campus-apartments are nicer.

3. **On Earth, _____ are seven continents.**

   A. their   C. theer

   B. there   D. they're

4. **Which word is an adverb that describes the underlined verb?**

   The man <u>spoke</u> to us wisely.

   A. man   C. us

   B. to   D. wisely

5. **What part of speech are the underlined words in the following sentence?**

   Twelve students passed the exam, <u>but</u> seven did not, <u>so</u> the teacher is letting them retake it.

   A. Adjective   C. Conjunction

   B. Preposition D. Adverb

6. **Which words in the following sentence are proper nouns?**

   Matthew had a meeting with his supervisor on Tuesday.

   A. Matthew, meeting

   B. Matthew, Tuesday

   C. meeting, supervisor

   D. supervisor, Tuesday

7. **Which pronoun correctly completes the following sentence?**

   Nigel introduced Van and ____ to the new administrator.

   A. I   C. she

   B. me   D. they

8. **Which of the following verbs correctly completes this sentence?**

   William didn't think he would enjoy the musical, but he ____.

   A. do   C. liked

   B. did   D. would

9. **How many verbs must agree with the underlined subject in the following sentence?**

   <u>Kareem Abdul-Jabbar</u>, my favorite basketball player, dribbles, shoots, and scores to win the game!

   A. 0   C. 2

   B. 1   D. 3

10. **Select the part of speech that is always in the predicate.**

    A. Noun   C. Adjective

    B. Pronoun   D. Verb

11. **Identify the dependent clause in the following sentence.**

When I lived in New York City, I took the subway to work every day.

A. When I lived in New York City

B. I took the subway

C. To work every day

D. In New York City

12. **Which of the following coordinating conjunctions correctly completes the following sentence?**

My daughter is in the school play, _____ I want to go to every performance.

A. so

B. or

C. but

D. and

13. **Which of the following options would complete the above sentence to make it a compound sentence?**

The class of middle school students

_____.

A. served food at

B. served food at a soup kitchen

C. served food at a soup kitchen, and they enjoyed the experience

D. served food at a soup kitchen even though they weren't required to

14. **Which of the following is an example of a compound sentence?**

A. Felix has taken Taekwondo for years, now he is a black belt.

B. Felix has taken Taekwondo for years and now he is a black belt.

C. Felix has taken Taekwondo for years, and now he is a black belt.

D. Felix has taken Taekwondo for years because now he is a black belt.

15. **Which of the following options would give the sentence below a parallel structure?**

The room was cleaned, painted and

_____.

A. Tory redecorated it

B. redecorated by Tory

C. redecorating by Tory

D. Tory as redecorating it

16. **Which of the following is an example of a complex sentence?**

A. Timothy got a massage after running.

B. After running, Timothy got a massage.

C. Since Timothy went running he got a massage.

D. Timothy went running, and then he got a massage.

17. **Which of the following sentences uses the MOST formal language?**

A. We connect blonde hair with silliness.

B. We believe blonde hair means silliness.

C. Blonde hair is often associated with silliness.

D. People think blonde hair means silliness.

18. **In which of the following situations would it be best to use informal language?**

A. A charity event

B. A football game

C. A job interview

D. A dentist's office

19. **Which of the following is the meaning of "jam" as used in this sentence?**

    The copy machine had a paper <u>jam</u>, and the technician had to come fix it.

    A. A backup in traffic

    B. An awkward situation or predicament

    C. An instance of a machine seizing or getting stuck

    D. An informal gathering of musicians improvising together

20. **Which of the following context clues correctly helps you define the word "solution" in this sentence?**

    Claude used a solution of ammonia and water to clean the mess that was on the floor.

    A. "Claude used"

    B. "ammonia and water"

    C. "to clean"

    D. "the floor"

21. **Which of the following is the meaning of "miserly" as used in this sentence?**

    The old man was <u>miserly</u>, and he rarely spent his money on anything.

    A. Stingy   C. Cranky

    B. Selfish   D. Uncaring

22. **Which of the following context clues correctly helps you define the word "boisterous" in this sentence?**

    The heavy metal concert had a <u>boisterous</u> crowd of fans who hooted and howled during the whole performance.

    A. "heavy metal concert"

    B. "crowd of fans"

    C. "hooted and howled"

    D. "whole performance"

23. **Which of the following is the meaning of "riot" as used in this sentence?**

    Agatha is an absolute <u>riot</u>, and people enjoy listening to her crazy stories.

    A. A large group of uncontrolled people

    B. A place filled with something

    C. Someone or something that is very funny

    D. An angry speech

24. **What is the best definition of the word** *egocentric?*

    A. Selfish   C. Focused

    B. Friendly   D. Resentful

25. **Which of the following suffixes means "full of"?**

    A. -er   C. -ness

    B. -en   D. -ous

26. **Which of the following root words means "to make"?**

    A. fac   C. fant

    B. fric   D. fract

27. Which of the following prefixes means "above"?

    A. sub-   C. inter-

    B. trans-   D. super-

28. The use of the root *mers* in the word *immerse* indicates which the following?

    A. Something is dipped in liquid.

    B. Something is heated in liquid.

    C. Something got sprayed with liquid.

    D. Something is kept away from liquid.

TEAS Practice Exam 2
Answer Key with Explanatory Answers

Section I. Reading

1. B. All of the sentences are related in some way to the text, but the topic is specifically about an account of human impact on an animal species. **Skill: Main Ideas, Topic Sentences, and Supporting Details.**

2. C. The best topic sentence to unite the information would be the one about human encroachment negatively impacting the koala population. The others would be additional supporting details. **Skill: Main Ideas, Topic Sentences, and Supporting Details.**

3. D. Each of the sentences is related in some way to the passage, but the detail about the number of koala pathways that have been built is the best fit for the topic of the text. **Skill: Main Ideas, Topic Sentences, and Supporting Details.**

4. A. Although the text mentions that a jack-o-lantern can rot once it is on display, this is not a step to follow in the process. Scooping out the pulp is one of the steps. **Skill: Summarizing Text and Using Text Features.**

5. B. The text states that drawing a design on the pumpkin helps prevent cutting errors. **Skill: Summarizing Text and Using Text Features.**

6. B. The words "Then" and "Next" indicate sequence because they tell you when to do a step. **Skill: Summarizing Text and Using Text Features.**

7. B. The prefix "pre" in the word "pre-greased" means "before," so the cookie sheet needs to be greased sometime before putting the batter onto it. **Skill: Summarizing Text and Using Text Features.**

8. B. Since this is the final step, you would use the word "last" to indicate it is the final step in the directions. **Skill: Summarizing Text and Using Text Features.**

9. C. The thesis is the point the author defends throughout the essay. In this case, it is the proposal to create butterfly habitat along the highways. **Skill: The Writing Process.**

10. C. Sentence 7 proposes changing the way highways are managed. Placing this sentence at the beginning of the paragraph would help link back to the thesis and show why the writer is sharing information about highway maintenance. **Skill: The Writing Process.**

11. A. The writer of this essay could highlight the link back to the main idea by mentioning pollinators or butterflies again in the opening sentence of the second body paragraph. **Skill: The Writing Process.**

12. C. Sentence 9 focuses on cost, so evidence to support it should also focus on costs. **Skill: The Writing Process.**

13. A. The quotation in sentence 11 is problematic in this draft because the speaker is not identified. **Skill: The Writing Process.**

14. B. Body paragraph 3 states that gardens need butterflies and other pollinators but does not develop the point or offer evidence to back it up. **Skill: The Writing Process.**

15. B. The conclusion should refer clearly back to the main point of the essay, which has not mentioned extinction. **Skill: The Writing Process.**

16. C. A call to action could make an effective ending to this essay because it would focus the reader on a specific, immediate plan rather than ending on an emotional point about an uncertain future. **Skill: The Writing Process.**

17. D. The first sentence of this paragraph should support the claim that J.K. Rowling expertly engages the audience's emotions. The sentence about readers feeling a kinship with Harry is the clearest and most direct link to this idea, so it belongs at the beginning. **Skill: Essay Revision and Transitions.**

18. B. As the paragraph explains, a third person limited omniscient narrator has access to one and only one character's thoughts. If the author shows a main character feeling surprised by another character's choices, the reader sees the main character's thoughts but only the supporting character's actions. **Skill: Essay Revision and Transitions.**

19. A. The transition *that is* interprets or clarifies a thought. This works in context because Sentence 2 clarifies the claim from Sentence 1 by explaining what it means. **Skill: Essay Revision and Transitions.**

20. A. Sentence 4 describes the consequence of the fact that readers cannot see into the minds of any character except Harry. This calls for a causation transition such as *therefore* or *thus*. **Skill: Essay Revision and Transitions.**

21. B. Any reasoning or explanation in an essay should stay closely focused on the point, explaining it in detail. Only the sentence about connecting emotionally with character's story does this. **Skill: Essay Revision and Transitions.**

22. C. This passage is an amusing description of an adolescent written by an adult who has enough experience to know that her daughter's huge emotions will pass and the little girl inside her will poke out. **Skill: Tone, Mood, and Transition Words.**

23. B. Authors use irony when their words do not literally mean what they say. The daughter is clearly having an awful day based on her words and actions, and the use of the word "marvelous" adds an ironic tone to the passage. **Skill: Tone, Mood, and Transition Words.**

24. A. This passage establishes irony in the opening sentence by applying a positive adjective, "celebratory," to an ordinary occurrence that is usually negative, such as the banging of a door. **Skill: Tone, Mood, and Transition Words.**

25. A. Effective readers would likely know this is just the life of an adolescent since we have all been through this time in our lives. Entertained would be a more likely reaction. **Skill: Tone, Mood, and Transition Words.**

26. A. The word "instantly" explains how quickly the mother felt "dismayed" but does not transition between ideas. **Skill: Tone, Mood, and Transition Words.**

27. B. "However" and "despite" both indicate a difference between ideas. **Skill: Tone, Mood, and Transition Words.**

28. B. "Furthermore" would be the transition to use as in: *Furthermore, she made a "tsk" sound.* This would show how the author is building on an established line of thought. **Skill: Tone, Mood, and Transition Words.**

29. C. The transition is the word that links the two ideas: *also*. **Skill: Tone, Mood, and Transition Words.**

30. C. Passage 1 is intended to persuade readers that termites are amazing insects. **Skill: Understanding Author's Purpose, Point of View, and Rhetorical Strategies.**

31. D. Passage 2 tells a story, which is meant to entertain. **Skill: Understanding Author's Purpose, Point of View, and Rhetorical Strategies.**

32. A. Passage 1 says, "Many people find termites to be destructive little pests, but they are actually ingenious little creatures." This suggests that termites are misunderstood and things are not always what they seem. **Skill: Understanding Author's Purpose, Point of View, and Rhetorical Strategies.**

33. B. The author of Passage 1 uses primarily facts and logic, although she could strengthen her points by clearly identifying sources or establishing her credentials. **Skill: Understanding Author's Purpose, Point of View, and Rhetorical Strategies.**

34. D. The techniques an author uses to support an argument or develop a main idea are called rhetorical strategies. **Skill: Understanding the Author's Purpose, Point of View, and Rhetorical Strategies.**

35. B. An author's point of view is a general outlook on the subject. **Skill: Understanding the Author's Purpose, Point of View, and Rhetorical Strategies.**

36. A. The main idea of a text is its key point, and the point of view is the author's outlook on the subject. The purpose is the reason for writing. **Skill: Understanding the Author's Purpose, Point of View, and Rhetorical Strategies.**

37. C. This passage shares the author's opinions about television and movie rating systems. This makes it a persuasive piece. **Skill: Understanding the Author's Purpose, Point of View, and Rhetorical Strategies.**

38. D. The author of the passage says that only she knows her kids well enough to be able to decide what they can watch. She would likely agree that other parents are the best people to make similar choices for their own kids. **Skill: Understanding the Author's Purpose, Point of View, and Rhetorical Strategies.**

39. C. The author of this passage suggests that parents should decide for themselves whether or not kids should watch certain shows or movies. She would likely agree with an effort to provide parents more information for making these choices. **Skill: Understanding the Author's Purpose, Point of View, and Rhetorical Strategies.**

40. D. The author includes her credentials as a parent to establish that she is a trustworthy authority on this subject. **Skill: Understanding the Author's Purpose, Point of View, and Rhetorical Strategies.**

41. D. A text feature is any element that stands out from the text, such as a title, a boldfaced section, or a graphic element. **Skill: Evaluating and Integrating Data.**

42. B. This passage argues that childhood obesity is a major problem in our country. **Skill: Facts, Opinions, and Evaluating an Argument.**

43. B. Factual information is verifiable and not based on personal beliefs or feelings. The statistic about the number of children who have been diagnosed as obese is a fact. **Skill: Facts, Opinions, and Evaluating an Argument.**

44. A. This statement takes a complex issue and presents it as if only two possible options are in play. This is an either/or fallacy. **Skill: Facts, Opinions, and Evaluating an Argument.**

45. C. The sentence in question is an example of circular reasoning. That is, it restates the argument in different words instead of providing evidence to back it up. **Skill: Facts, Opinions, and Evaluating an Argument.**

46. A. The phrase "very overweight" in this sentence reflects a judgment that is subject to interpretation. This indicates that the sentence reflects a belief rather than a fact. **Skill: Facts, Opinions, and Evaluating an Argument.**

47. A. Unlike an opinion, a fact is verifiably true. An argument or claim may express a fact, an opinion, or a mixture of the two. **Skill: Facts Opinions and Evaluating an Argument.**

48. D. Primary sources are written by people who witnessed the original creation or discovery of the information they present. An interview would be an example of a primary source. **Skill: Understanding Primary Sources, Making Inferences, and Drawing Conclusions.**

49. A. This author is not very trustworthy, but he does not make any attempt to conceal the fact that he is sharing his personal opinions rather than facts. The fact that he begins with the sentence "You know what I hate?" is a clear cue that this is argumentative writing. **Skill: Understanding Primary Sources, Making Inferences, and Drawing Conclusions.**

50. C. The sentence about freelancers not making as much money is one of the few logical points this blog post makes, but the writer does not share his sources. This makes it difficult for the reader to verify the information. **Skill: Understanding Primary Sources, Making Inferences, and Drawing Conclusions.**

51. B. The passage raises the opposing argument that freelancing provides greater freedom for workers, but the writer does not respond to this argument. Instead, he makes a manipulatively emotional argument. **Skill: Understanding Primary Sources, Making Inferences, and Drawing Conclusions.**

52. C. A government website tracking statistics might be a good source, but it would provide facts rather than opinions. An opinion article by an expert in the field would more likely offer what the student is looking for. **Skill: Understanding Primary Sources, Making Inferences, and Drawing Conclusions.**

53. C. In contrast with a moral, which is explicitly stated, a theme is a suggested, or implicit, deeper meaning behind a text. **Skill: Types of Passages, Text Structures, Genre and Theme.**

Section II. Mathematics

1. C. The correct solution is 2016 because there were 155 total participants. **Skill: Interpreting Graphics.**

2. D. The bill will cost $45.14 because the tip is equal to $8.14 since $37 × 0.22 = $8.14 + $37 bill = $45.14 total cost. **Skill: Ratios, Proportions, and Percentages.**

3. C. The older sibling answered 112 questions right because $\frac{60 \text{ correct}}{75 \text{ questions}} = \frac{X}{140 \text{ questions}}$ and $x = 112$ questions. **Skill: Ratios, Proportions, and Percentages.**

4. A. The correct solution is $\frac{3}{8}$ because $\frac{0.375}{1} = \frac{375}{1000} = \frac{3}{8}$. **Skill: Decimals and Fractions.**

5. B. The correct solution is 20.48 because 39.45−18.97 = 20.48 feet. **Skill: Solving Real World Mathematical Problems.**

6. B. The woman will have $4,336.50 because the annual interest will earn her $136.50. $4,200 × 0.0325 = $136.50 + $4,200 = $4,336.50. **Skill: Ratios, Proportions, and Percentages.**

7. A. The correct solution is $\frac{37}{40}$ because $\frac{1}{8} + \frac{4}{5} = \frac{5}{40} + \frac{32}{40} = \frac{5+32}{40} = \frac{37}{40}$. **Skill: Addition and Subtraction of Fractions.**

8. C. Either set up a proportion or just note that this question is asking for a fraction of a specific number: 15% (or $\frac{3}{20}$) of 64. Multiply $\frac{3}{20}$ by 64 to get $\frac{48}{5}$, or 48:5. **Skill: Ratios, Proportions, and Percentages.**

9. D. The correct solution is 48.6 because 5.4(3)(3) = 48.6 gallons. **Skill: Solving Real World Mathematical Problems.**

10. C. This problem can be solved by dividing the distance the mom must drive by the time she has available. (18 miles ÷ 20 minutes) × 60 minutes in an hour = 54 mph. **Skill: Solving Real World Mathematical Problems.**

11. B. The correct solution is $2\frac{1}{6}$ because $1\frac{1}{2} + \frac{2}{3} = \frac{3}{2} + \frac{2}{3} = \frac{9}{6} + \frac{4}{6} = \frac{13}{6} = 2\frac{1}{6}$. **Skill: Addition and Subtraction of Fractions.**

12. D. The event sponsors can give $2,000 to each volunteer because 320 × $75 = $24,000 ÷ 12 volunteers = $2,000 each. **Skill: Solving Real World Mathematical Problems.**

13. D. The correct solution is the difference between the maximum and minimum is 70 sales. The maximum value is 90, and the minimum value is 20. The difference between these values is 70 sales. **Skill: Interpreting Categorical and Quantitative Data.**

14. C. The correct solution is 4 because 6^2 = 36 − 4 = 32 ÷ 8 = 4. **Skill: Equations with One Variable.**

15. D. The correct solution is $y^3 - 4y^2 + 9y + 3$.

$$(3y^3 - 4y^2 + 6y + 3) - (2y^3 - 3y) = (3y^3 - 4y^2 + 6y + 3) + (-2y^3 + 3y)$$
$$= (3y^3 - 2y^3) - 4y^2 + (6y + 3y) + 3 = y^3 - 4y^2 + 9y + 3$$

Skill: Polynomials.

16. A. The taxi fare will cost $61.90 because $8.00 + ($3.85 × 14 miles) = $61.90, therefore the equation can be represented as $8.00 + 3.85m$ = $61.90. **Skill: Solving Real World Mathematical Problems.**

17. D. The correct solution is 750 grams. $0.75\ kg \times \frac{1,000\ g}{1\ kg} = 750\ g$. **Skill: Standards of Measure.**

18. D. The correct answer is $\frac{29}{35}$ because $\frac{29}{10} \div \frac{7}{2} = \frac{29}{10} \times \frac{2}{7} = \frac{58}{70} = \frac{29}{35}$. **Skill: Multiplication and Division of Fractions.**

19. D. The student earned a 71% on the exam because $\frac{125}{175} = \frac{5}{7} = 71\%$. **Skill: Ratios, Proportions, and Percentages.**

20. D. The correct solution is $2\frac{1}{2}$ because $2\frac{0.5}{1} = 2\frac{5}{10} = 2\frac{1}{2}$. **Skill: Decimals and Fractions.**

21. B. Samantha could run 10 kilometers in approximately 63 minutes because $\frac{50\ minutes}{8\ kilometers} = \frac{X}{10\ kilometers}$ and x = 62.5 minutes, rounded up to 63 minutes. **Skill: Ratios, Proportions, and Percentages.**

22. C. The correct solution is 10.8 because $A = \frac{1}{2}\pi r^2; 45 = \left(\frac{1}{2}\right)3.14\,r^2; 45 = 1.57\,r^2 = 28.66 = r^2$; $r \approx 5.4$. The diameter is twice the radius, or about 10.8 centimeters. **Skill: Circles.**

23. C. The correct solution is 9.84 yards. $9\text{ m} \times \frac{3.28\text{ ft}}{1\text{ m}} \times \frac{1\text{ yd}}{3\text{ ft}} = \frac{29.52}{3} = 9.84$ yd. **Skill: Standards of Measure.**

24. B. The correct solution is $12.50 because she worked a total of $4.25(2) + 6.5(2) = 8.5 + 13 = 21.5$ hours. The hourly rate is $268.75 \div 21.50 = \$12.50$. **Skill: Solving Real World Mathematical Problems.**

25. C. The correct solution 12 units. The difference between the x-coordinates is $6-(-6) = 12$ units and the difference between the y-coordinates is $6-(-6) = 12$ units. **Skill: Similarity, Right Triangles, and Trigonometry.**

26. A. The correct solution is 32.73 kilograms. $72\text{ lb} \times \frac{1\text{ kg}}{2.2\text{ lb}} = \frac{72}{2.2} = 32.73$ kg. **Skill: Standards of Measure.**

27. B. The correct solution is 3. Substitute the values into the formula $54 = 6s^2$. Solve the equation by dividing both sides of the equation by 6 and applying the square root, $9 = s^2; s = 3$ feet. **Skill: Similarity, Right Triangles, and Trigonometry.**

28. D. The difference between Logan's salary is 75 cents because $10.25 - $9.50 = $0.75. Setting up a proportion reveals that 75 cents of an originally $9.50 an hour salary is a 7.9% increase. **Skill: Ratios, Proportions, and Percentages.**

29. B. The correct solution is –2.

$6x = -12$ — Add 12 to both sides of the equation.
$x = -2$ — Divide both sides of the equation by 6.

Skill: Equations with One Variable.

30. D. The correct answer is $2\frac{31}{42}$ because $\frac{23}{14} \div \frac{3}{5} = \frac{23}{14} \times \frac{5}{3} = \frac{115}{42} = 2\frac{31}{42}$. **Skill: Multiplication and Division of Fractions.**

31. C. The correct answer is $11.\overline{1}\%$ because $0.\overline{1}$ as a percent is $0.\overline{1} \times 100 = 11.\overline{1}\%$. **Skill: Decimals and Fractions.**

32. B. If 1 out of every 250 contract a disease, the fraction of people is $\frac{1}{250}$, which is equal to 0.004. Multiply by 100% to get 0.4%. **Skill: Ratios, Proportions, and Percentages.**

33. C. The correct solution is 6 because the equation simplifies to $4x = 25 - 1 = 24$ and $x = 6$. **Skill: Equations with One Variable.**

34. C. The correct solution is $\frac{4}{3}$.

$$3x = 4 \qquad \text{Subtract 8 from both sides of the equation.}$$
$$x = \frac{4}{3} \qquad \text{Divide both sides of the equation by 3.}$$

Skill: Equations with One Variable.

35. C. The correct solution is May to June because the increase is 20 cars, which is the largest. **Skill: Interpreting Graphics.**

36. D. The correct solution is less than half of the children like fish, rabbits, or birds. There are 85 children who like cats or dogs. There are 55 children who like fish, rabbits, or birds, which is less than half. **Skill: Interpreting Categorical and Quantitative Data.**

Section III. Science

1. D. The transverse plane is parallel to the surface of the ground and divides the body into superior and inferior planes. **Skill: Organization of the Human Body.**

2. B. The ventral cavity contains the abdominal, pelvic, and thoracic cavities. **Skill: Organization of the Human Body.**

3. A. Blood flows in one direction when it leaves the aorta and travels through the arteries. **Skill: Cardiovascular System.**

4. C. The buffy coat, found between the reddish mass and liquid plasma of blood, consists of leukocytes, or white blood cells. **Skill: Cardiovascular System.**

5. D. Age does not significantly affect thyroid hormones. **Skill: Endocrine System.**

6. C. Both luteinizing hormones and follicle-stimulating hormones promote sperm cell production in males. **Skill: Endocrine System.**

7. A. Each hormone can only bind to its receptor molecules and cannot influence the function of cells that do not have receptor molecules for the hormone. **Skill: Endocrine System.**

8. B. Lipase is an enzyme that breaks down lipids. **Skill: Gastrointestinal System.**

9. C. One of the functions of the pancreas is to release bicarbonate ions, which neutralize acids. **Skill: Gastrointestinal System.**

10. C. Pepsin is an enzyme produced in the stomach which breaks down proteins as they enter. **Skill: Gastrointestinal System.**

11. A. Tanning beds and overexposure to the sun are common sources of UV radiation. UVA and UVB rays are known to cause skin cancer in people. **Skill: Integumentary System.**

12. B. Hair is an accessory organ that insulates the body. The hair on a person's head traps heat to help maintain the body's temperature. **Skill: Integumentary System.**

13. D. Epidermal cells are found deep in the stratum basale. From there, they travel to the skin's surface, producing keratin along the way. This keratin creates the waterproof layer, or stratum corneum. **Skill: Integumentary System.**

14. C. The tonsils, adenoids, and appendix were believed to be vestigial organs. The spleen was never considered vestigial. **Skill: The Lymphatic System.**

15. C. The immune system sometimes does its job too well and mounts a major defense against a harmless substance. Such an immune system response is called an allergy. **Skill: The Lymphatic System.**

16. C. The thymus gland secretes hormones that stimulate the maturation of the killer T cells. It is active from birth through puberty. **Skill: The Lymphatic System.**

17. B. The B cells label invaders for later destruction by macrophages. **Skill: The Lymphatic System.**

18. C. Ligaments are structures that attach bone to bone. They allow less movement than other structures like joints. **Skill: Muscular System.**

19. D. All muscles contract following stimulation by the nervous system, as in the case of skeletal muscles, or from stimulation by both the nervous system and circulating hormones, in the case of smooth and cardiac muscles. **Skill: Muscular System.**

20. D. The cell membrane that surrounds a muscle fiber is the sarcolemma. Within this sarcolemma is the cytoplasm of the cell, called the sarcoplasm. **Skill: Muscular System.**

21. A. The peripheral nervous system is divided into the somatic and autonomic nervous systems. The autonomic nervous system transmits neural signals to the smooth muscle found in the walls of internal organs and structures like blood vessels. **Skill: The Nervous System.**

22. C. The cell body, or soma, contains the nucleus of the neuron. Inside the nucleus is DNA, which contains the genetic information for the neuron. Other organelles are also found inside the cell body. **Skill: The Nervous System.**

23. C. Smell is the only sense that bypasses the thalamus during external signal processing by the CNS. The thalamus is the structure of the limbic system that directly receives sensory information from nerves. **Skill: The Nervous System.**

24. A. The basic human body plan is developed by the end of embryogenesis. At this stage, not all organs and systems are entirely functional, but the basic pattern and structure are complete. It is elaborated throughout gestation, and some changes occur during puberty. **Skill: Reproductive System.**

25. C. The ova (egg cells) and sperm are female and male haploid gametes, respectively, and are analogs. **Skill: Reproductive System.**

26. D. The diaphragm is a muscle that plays a role in breathing. When a person exhales, carbon dioxide is removed from the body. This happens as air is pushed out of the lungs when the diaphragm relaxes. **Skill: The Respiratory System.**

27. C. The diaphragm is a muscle that is found at the base of the lungs and across the bottom of the rib cage. **Skill: The Respiratory System.**

28. C. The appendicular skeleton consists of bones that belong to the upper and lower extremities, such as the pelvic girdle. This bone is found at the base of the vertebral column where the femur attaches. **Skill: Skeletal System.**

29. D. The flat bone is a broad, thin bone that is the site for muscle attachment in the body to aid in movement. Examples of this bone are the hipbone and scapula. **Skill: Skeletal System.**

30. B. There are five types of bone in the human body: long bone, short bone, irregular bone, sesamoid bone, and flat bone. **Skill: Skeletal System.**

31. C. Roughly 180 liters of blood leave the renal artery on a daily basis, enter the glomerulus in the nephrons, and proceed through the renal tubules. The byproduct of this fluid, which is urine, empties into the bladder for storage. **Skill: The Urinary System.**

32. A. Urine is a byproduct of the blood that is filtered in the kidneys. This tubular filtrate travels to the ureter, which is a muscular tube that contracts to push urine to the urethra and out of the body. **Skill: The Urinary System.**

33. B. In the molecular structure of water, a partially negative oxygen atom is bonded to two partially positive hydrogen atoms. **Skill: An Introduction to Biology.**

34. A. Lipids are a class of biomolecules that provide a long-term storage solution for energy in living things. Examples of lipids include fats, steroids, and oils. **Skill: An Introduction to Biology.**

35. D. Ribosomes are organelles that play a role in the synthesis of proteins such as enzymes. **Skill: Cell Structure, Function, and Type.**

36. D. An animal cell is a eukaryotic cell, which means it lacks a flagellum. Unlike plant cells, which have chloroplasts and a cell wall, animal cells contain a Golgi apparatus. **Skill: Cell Structure, Function, and Type.**

37. B. After DNA replicates, it wraps around proteins called histones to form a chromosome. The chromosome must be formed for mitosis to occur. **Skill: Cellular Reproduction, Cellular Respiration, and Photosynthesis.**

38. B. During the electron transport chain, chemiosmosis occurs. This happens when electrons and protons from NADH are released to generate large amounts of ATP. **Skill: Cellular Reproduction, Cellular Respiration, and Photosynthesis.**

39. A. ATP and NADH are produced are produced during the light reactions of photosynthesis. During the dark reactions, these organic molecules are used to create sugar molecules. **Skill: Cellular Reproduction, Cellular Respiration, and Photosynthesis.**

40. D. Each nucleotide has three parts: a five-carbon sugar molecule, a phosphate group, and a nitrogen base. **Skill: Genetics and DNA.**

41. A. Translation produces short sequences of proteins called amino acids. **Skill: Genetics and DNA.**

42. C. The process that rewrites the information in a gene in DNA into a molecule of messenger RNA is called transcription. **Skill: Genetics and DNA.**

43. B. One of the alleles is dominant, so it is expressed. **Skill: Genetics and DNA.**

44. D. Researchers must use inductive and deductive reasoning to formulate a plausible ... **Designing an Experiment.**

... type of car used during the experiment is not manipulated, this is a type of ... **igning an Experiment.**

... ositive correlation between bird migration and time. As time increases, the ... bird travels also increases. **Skill: Designing an Experiment.**

... **D.** For an atom to carry a negative charge, it must have more negatively charged electrons than positively charged protons. **Skill: Scientific Notation.**

48. D. Magnesium and aluminum are the only pair located in the same period (row) of the periodic table, period 3. **Skill: Scientific Notation.**

49. C. This silver isotope has a mass number of 109. Silver has 47 protons, which contribute 47 to the mass number. To get the number of neutrons, subtract: $109 - 47 = 62$. This atom contains 62 neutrons. **Skill: Scientific Notation.**

50. D. In the lungs, oxygen diffuses into the bloodstream because there is a higher concentration of oxygen molecules in the lungs' air sacs than there is in the blood. **Skill: Properties of Matter.**

51. D. Magnesium and chlorine are balanced, but hydrogen is not. In the unbalanced equation, there are two atoms of hydrogen in the reactants and four atoms of hydrogen in the products. The student has placed an unnecessary coefficient in front of H_2. See the balanced equation below. **Skill: Chemical Equations.**

$$Mg + 2HCl \rightarrow MgCl_2 + H_2$$

52. B. The goal of diffusion is for molecules to reach equilibrium in an area. **Skill: Properties of Matter.**

53. D. Evidence of a chemical property is that a new substance—in this case, rust—is formed. **Skill: Properties of Matter.**

Section IV. English and Language Usage

1. C. *Gone with the Wind.* Publication titles are capitalized. Shorter prepositions, articles, and conjunctions within titles are not capitalized. **Skill: Capitalization.**

2. C. *Off-campus apartments are nicer.* Hyphens are often used for compound words that are placed before the noun to help with understanding. **Skill: Punctuation.**

3. B. *There* describes a place or position and is correctly spelled. **Skill: Spelling.**

4. D. *Wisely* is an adverb that describes the verb *spoke.* **Skill: Adjectives and Adverbs.**

5. C. *But* and *so* are coordinating conjunctions. These two conjunctions connect three independent clauses in this sentence. **Skill: Conjunctions and Prepositions.**

6. B. *Matthew* and *Tuesday* are proper nouns. **Skill: Nouns.**

7. B. An object pronoun must be used here. **Skill: Pronouns.**

8. B. *Did* can be used here, for a shortened form of *did enjoy it.* **Skill: Verbs and Verb Tenses.**

9. D. The verbs *dribbles, shoots,* and *scores* must agree with the subject *Kareem Abdul-Jabbar.* **Skill: Subject and Verb Agreement.**

10. D. The predicate is the part of the sentence that contains the verb. **Skill: Subject and Verb Agreement.**

11. A. When I lived in New York City. It is dependent because it does not express a complete thought and relies on the independent clause. The word "when" also signifies the beginning of a dependent clause. **Skill: Types of Clauses.**

12. A. *So.* It is the only conjunction that fits within the context of the sentence. **Skill: Types of Clauses.**

13. C. This option would make the sentence a compound sentence. **Skill: Types of Sentences.**

14. C. This is a compound sentence joining two independent clauses with a comma and the conjunction *and.* **Skill: Types of Sentences.**

15. B. *Redecorated by Tory* would be parallel in structure since the list begins in passive voice and uses the past tense of the verbs. **Skill: Types of Sentences.**

16. B. This is a complex sentence because it starts with a subordinating conjunction, *after*, has a dependent clause followed by a comma, and then has an independent clause. **Skill: Types of Sentences.**

17. C. Blonde hair is often associated with silliness. The sentence is the most formal because it does not use pronouns and has more formal vocabulary. **Skill: Formal and Informal Language.**

18. B. A football game. A stadium is an informal setting where formal language is not necessary. **Skill: Formal and Informal Language.**

19. C. The meaning of jam in the context of this sentence is "an instance of a machine seizing or getting stuck." **Skill: Context Clues and Multiple Meaning Words.**

20. B. The meaning of solution in this context is "a mixture of two or more substances." The phrase "ammonia and water" helps you figure out which meaning of solution is being used. **Skill: Context Clues and Multiple Meaning Words.**

21. A. The meaning of miserly in the context of this sentence is "stingy." **Skill: Context Clues and Multiple Meaning Words.**

22. C. The meaning of boisterous in this context is "noisy and active in a lively way." The phrase "hooted and howled" helps you figure out the meaning of boisterous. **Skill: Context Clues and Multiple Meaning Words.**

23. C. The meaning of riot in the context of this sentence is "someone or something that is very funny." **Skill: Context Clues and Multiple Meaning Words.**

24. A. The root *ego* means "self," so *egocentric* means "selfish." **Skill: Root Words, Prefixes, and Suffixes.**

25. B. The suffix that means "full of" is *-en* as in the word *golden*. **Skill: Root Words, Prefixes, and Suffixes.**

26. A. The root that means "to make" is *fac* as in the word *manufacture*. **Skill: Root Words, Prefixes, and Suffixes.**

27. D. The prefix that means "above" is *super-* as in the word *supervisor*. **Skill: Root Words, Prefixes, and Suffixes.**

28. A. The root *mers* means "dip or dive," so *immerse* indicates that something is dipped in liquid. **Skill: Root Words, Prefixes, and Suffixes.**

TEAS PRACTICE EXAM 3

SECTION I. READING

You have 64 minutes to complete 53 questions.

Read the following paragraph and answer questions 1-2.

Faith sighed as the old lady cooed at the baby and blabbed about her own children's early days. Four kids! They all walked and talked early! They were little geniuses! Blah blah blah! Faith spent twenty-four hours a day caring for a drooling, incontinent little person, and as a reward she had to hear constant stories about *other* drooling, incontinent little people. Maybe she should take a tip from the baby and erupt into a random fit of screaming.

1. **What is the topic sentence of the paragraph?**

   A. Maybe she should take a tip from the baby and erupt in a random fit of screaming.

   B. Faith spent twenty hours a day caring for a drooling, incontinent little person, and as a reward she had to hear four million stories about *other* drooling, incontinent little people.

   C. Faith sighed as the old lady cooed at the baby and blabbed about her own children's early days.

   D. None of the above; the main idea is implied.

2. **Which sentence best expresses the main idea of the paragraph?**

   A. Faith regrets that she ever became a mother and wishes she could give her baby up for adoption.

   B. Faith dislikes cleaning up drool and changing diapers, and she thinks the old lady is a liar or a fool.

   C. Faith feels frustrated when people bother her with nostalgic reminiscences about caring for small children.

   D. Faith is an unpleasant person with no empathy for lonely old ladies who desperately need to talk to someone.

Please read the text below and answer questions 3-7.

Desserts are known as the "forbidden food" in most diets. But dark chocolate is a sweet that people can enjoy because of its undeniable health benefits. Categorized as an "antioxidant," dark chocolate is known to fight free radicals, the unbalanced compounds created by cellular processes that can harm the body. This amazing sweet treat is also known to lower blood pressure, improve blood flow, and reduce heart disease risk in people. Studies have shown that dark chocolate can even improve people's brain function. There is considerable evidence that dark chocolate can provide powerful benefits, but it is still loaded with calories, so consuming too much is not recommended. People can reap the benefits of dark chocolate by eating it in moderation.

3. **The topic of this paragraph is:**

   A. foods that battle heart disease.

   B. healthy dessert recipes.

   C. cooking with dark chocolate.

   D. benefits of dark chocolate.

4. **The topic sentence of this paragraph is:**

   A. Desserts are known as the "forbidden food" in most diets.

   B. But dark chocolate is a sweet that people can enjoy because of its undeniable health benefits.

   C. This amazing sweet treat is also known to lower blood pressure, improve blood flow, and reduce heart disease risk in people.

   D. People can reap the benefits of dark chocolate by eating it in moderation.

5. **If the author added a description of a popular recipe using dark chocolate as its main ingredient, what type of information would this be?**

   A. A main idea

   B. A topic sentence

   C. A supporting detail

   D. An off-topic sentence

6. **Read the following description of the paragraph:**

   The author fails to offer a holistic view of dark chocolate by only presenting its benefits and never exploring its downsides.

   Why is this *not* a valid description of the main idea?

   A. It is not accurate; the author of the paragraph is stating facts, not opinions.

   B. It is not objective; the person summarizing the main idea is biased since he/she is in the medical field.

   C. It is not accurate; the author of the paragraph does warn the reader to eat dark chocolate in moderation.

   D. It is not objective; the person summarizing the main idea is obviously not a fan of dark chocolate.

7. **Why isn't a statistic about how much chocolate is consumed on a daily basis by the average American suitable for this passage?**

   A. It does not directly support the main idea that dark chocolate is good for your health.

   B. Readers might feel the author is passing judgment on how much chocolate Americans consume.

   C. Statistics should never be used as supporting details in persuasive writing.

   D. It would act as a second topic sentence and confuse readers about the main idea.

Read the following text and then answer questions 8-10.

In the late morning, Cynthia met Max at the state park where he had been waiting. They went on a hike. They followed a path that first led them through the deep, lush woods. The path then took them past a beautiful, serene lake. They were beginning to get thirsty, so they stopped to sit on a large rock to drink some water. Next, they continued hiking and came upon a clearing, Cynthia was astonished to see a picnic blanket all set up with plates and a picnic basket.

"Max!" she exclaimed.

Max had set up the picnic to surprise Cynthia.

8. **According to the paragraph, which event happened first?**

   A. Cynthia met Max at a state park in the late morning.

   B. Max set up the picnic for him and Cynthia.

   C. Cynthia and Max walked past a lake.

   D. Cynthia and Max stopped to drink water on a rock.

9. **Which word clues help you understand that this event happened first?**

   A. "had set up"

   B. "first went"

   C. "beginning to get"

   D. "in the late morning"

10. **Which of the following words from the passage is *not* a sequence word?**

   A. First   C. Next

   B. Then   D. Beginning

Read the paragraph below and answer questions 11-12.

H.D.'s poem "Oread" creates a metaphorical connection between the sea and the land. In the opening lines of the poem, she writes, "Whirl up, sea—/ whirl your pointed pines." The "pointed pines" in these lines are waves.

11. **This paragraph would be improved if the author:**

   A. stated a reason for choosing H.D.'s poetry as a topic.

   B. identified the source of the quotation in the second sentence.

   C. explained the connection between the point and the evidence.

   D. defined the word *metaphor* to prove an understanding of the term.

12. **Which sentence most naturally completes the thought developed in this paragraph?**

   A. The poet is using apostrophe when she addresses the sea directly as she would a person.

   B. The repetition of *p* sounds in this phrase is an example of a poetic technique called alliteration.

   C. H.D. does not call the waves by their real name because she wants the reader to think she is describing a forest.

   D. By comparing waves to trees, H.D. blurs the distinction between the wild ocean and the solid shore.

13. What is a mind map?

    A. A linear arrangement of ideas

    B. An associative arrangement of ideas

    C. The step before editing in the writing process

    D. The step after prewriting in the writing process

14. Revising is:

    A. fixing mechanical errors.

    B. making a plan for writing.

    C. getting the first draft down.

    D. improving content and structure.

15. Notes about source materials within a text are called:

    A. citations.

    B. research.

    C. revisions.

    D. mind maps.

16. Which strategy is recommended during the drafting phase?

    A. List all ideas that come to mind without worrying whether they're good or on-topic.

    B. Don't worry about noting where you got your information; save that step for the end.

    C. Stop writing frequently to look up grammar rules and words you don't know how to spell.

    D. Get the ideas down on paper, even if some sentences sound awkward or contain errors.

Read the following draft essay and answer questions 17-24.

Last week I saw a bad television commercial. (1) It said that women need more "self-confidence," and that breast augmentation surgery can give it to them. (2) I do not think plastic surgery leads to self-confidence. (3) True self-confidence comes from the belief in our accomplishments, not from the belief that we look good. (4)

Our society sends the message that women need to look like fashion models, but fashion models' body types aren't normal. (5) Many suffer from anorexia, and some have undergone plastic surgery to conform to a false ideal of beauty. (6) And what is the point of aiming for that unattainable ideal? (7) It takes time and energy that could be focused on more important matters. (8)

Women are told they need to look perfect, but nobody actually looks perfect. (9) Even the pictures in magazines are airbrushed and augmented. (10) They are not real. (11) And the women in those pictures are unusually pretty, plus they have professional help to keep their bodies looking as close to our false ideal of beauty as possible. (12) Ordinary women who have to spend time working every day and caring for their families have no chance of attaining anything close to that level of beauty. (13)

If you're like me, you may feel a pressure to measure up to society's false ideal of beauty. (14) But you shouldn't. (15) As women, we need to focus on making the world better, not on making our faces prettier. (16)

17. The word *bad* in Sentence 1 is poor word choice because it is not:

A. simple.

B. precise.

C. positive.

D. inclusive.

18. Which revision of Sentence 1 leads the reader more precisely toward the author's main idea?

A. Last week I saw a television commercial that left me outraged.

B. Last week I saw a television commercial that should be banned.

C. Last week I saw a commercial that was not aiming to sell anything.

D. Last week I saw a poorly acted and directed television commercial.

19. If Sentence 4 is the thesis statement, which statement accurately expresses a problem the writer should address in revision?

A. The thesis has nothing to do with television.

B. The thesis contains spelling and grammar errors.

C. The body paragraphs do not clearly defend the thesis.

D. The thesis directly contradicts the conclusion paragraph.

20. Which thesis statement should replace Sentence 4 to align more clearly with the points the author makes in the body of the essay?

A. The media's ideal of beauty cannot be achieved.

B. Fashion models are often victims of eating disorders.

C. More women need to get involved in business and politics.

D. Television commercials about breast augmentation should be banned.

21. Re-read the topic sentences of the two body paragraphs:

Our society sends the message that women need to look like fashion models, but fashion models' body types aren't normal. (Sentence 5)

Women are told they need to look perfect, but nobody actually looks perfect. (Sentence 9)

In revision, the author needs to address the fact that these two sentences:

A. contradict each other.

B. make the same basic point.

C. advocate for plastic surgery.

D. stereotype the fashion industry.

22. The author of this essay wants to add a body paragraph claiming that most women spend too much time and money trying to look good. Which evidence would *not* help support this point?

    A. Descriptions of expensive beauty products available at the local drug store

    B. Quotations from women admitting they sacrifice sleep to spend time on make-up

    C. Statistics about the amount of money women spend on clothes and beauty items

    D. Examples of women who minimize their beauty routines to maximize efficiency at work

23. Which transition word *best* fits at the beginning of Sentence 3?

    A. Moreover

    B. Therefore

    C. Personally

    D. Inconsequentially

24. Which revision to Sentence 5 would make the word choice more appropriately formal for an academic essay?

    A. Delete the phrase *body types.*

    B. Replace *aren't* with *are not.*

    C. Change *women* to *human beings.*

    D. Eliminate the reference to models.

25. Readers can determine tone primarily by examining:

    A. setting.   C. their feelings.

    B. word choice.   D. connecting words.

26. Which term refers to the feelings a text creates in the reader?

    A. Tone   C. Mood

    B. Irony   D. Theme

27. The tone of a text is:

    A. a word or phrase that links ideas.

    B. the reader's emotional response.

    C. a structural pattern in a series of words.

    D. the author's attitude toward the subject.

Read the following text and answer questions 28-31.

Our survey revealed some eye-opening results about young people and the role technology plays in their lives: technology is the primary focus of young people today. In our survey, 85% of those questioned said they spend their free time using technology in some way. Only 5% claim that they read actual books, 7% hang out with friends, and only 3% do some sort of physical activity. Whether it's looking through social media sites, playing video games, texting friends, or surfing the web, our youth spends an inordinate amount of time on screens. The days of hanging with friends, being outside in nature, and reading a good book for fun seem to be long gone.

Natalie Greenburg, clinical psychologist from the Perkins Institute, claims that, "Studies have shown a direct correlation between too much screen time and rising depression rates among teens." Greenburg explains screen time has an impact on how individuals view themselves. This is based on the amount of likes someone gets on social media sites or the number of texts someone receives from his or her peers. "The feedback kids get from technology becomes the barometer for their self-worth, which could lead to depression." Cyber bullying is also a big issue with technology. "Kids are able to freely say anything they want behind a screen," Greenburg states, "Since they are bullying from a keyboard, kids are no longer exposed to social cues like facial expressions and body language, which may stop the behavior. As a result, cyber bullying has become rampant, which has led to more depression."

Technology is here to stay and it is only going to become more entrenched in our society. It will continue to impact our youth in ways we can't even fathom.

28. **What is the primary purpose of the passage?**

   A. To inform   C. To persuade

   B. To caution   D. To entertain

29. **With which statement would the author of the passage most likely agree?**

   A. Technology is having a negative impact on our youth.

   B. Technology will eventually become obsolete.

   C. Technology will change for the better in the near future.

   D. Technology provides our youth with endless possibilities.

30. **Which sentence would express an additional effective reason to support the main idea of this passage?**

   A. Every teacher feels technology is getting in the way of classroom learning.

   B. A recent screen time study shows that technology use has risen since it is available in so many forms.

   C. Everyone feels young people have no hope since they are too dependent on technology.

   D. All young people know they are more technologically savvy than their parents will ever be.

31. **The author most likely included Natalie Greenburg's comments in order to:**

   A. explain the effects that technology is having on young people.

   B. add an emotional component to the statistical information presented.

   C. appeal to the reader's reason by adding statistical data to back up an opinion.

   D. distract readers by tricking them into believing the argument is not sufficiently supported.

32. **What is the most likely purpose of a science fiction book about genetic mutants waging war against human beings?**

   A. To decide   C. To persuade

   B. To inform   D. To entertain

Consider the following chart and answer the questions 33-34.

Infant Length-for-Age Chart, Female

Age (in months)	3rd Percentile Length (in centimeters)	5th Percentile Length (in centimeters)	10th Percentile Length (in centimeters)	25th Percentile Length (in centimeters)	50th Percentile Length (in centimeters)	75th Percentile Length (in centimeters)	90th Percentile Length (in centimeters)	95th Percentile Length (in centimeters)	97th Percentile Length (in centimeters)
0	45.09488	45.57561	46.33934	47.68345	49.2864	51.0187	52.7025	53.77291	54.49527
0.5	47.46916	47.96324	48.74248	50.09686	51.68358	53.36362	54.96222	55.96094	56.62728
1.5	50.95701	51.47996	52.29627	53.69078	55.28613	56.93136	58.45612	59.38911	60.00338
2.5	53.62925	54.17907	55.03144	56.47125	58.09382	59.74045	61.24306	62.15166	62.74547
3.5	55.8594	56.43335	57.31892	58.80346	60.45981	62.1233	63.62648	64.52875	65.11577
4.5	57.8047	58.40032	59.31633	60.84386	62.5367	64.22507	65.74096	66.64653	67.23398
5.5	59.54799	60.16323	61.10726	62.6759	64.40633	66.12418	67.65995	68.57452	69.16668
6.5	61.13893	61.77208	62.7421	64.35005	66.11842	67.8685	69.42868	70.35587	70.95545

33. The value in the bottom-right corner of this chart is 70.95545. This number represents:

   A. the length of a baby who is not yet 6.5 months old.

   B. the length of a baby who is closer to 6.9 months old.

   C. the length of a 6.5-month-old baby in the 97th percentile.

   D. the length of a baby who is closer to the 99th percentile.

34. At 2.5 months, Candice is 63.5 centimeters long. Which statement about her length is correct?

   A. It is about average for babies her age.

   B. It is between the 95th and 97th percentile for babies her age.

   C. It is above the 97th percentile for babies her age.

   D. It is incorrect; babies her age cannot be longer than about 62.75 centimeters.

35. What is the most likely purpose of an article that claims some genetic research is immoral?

   A. To decide   C. To persuade

   B. To inform   D. To entertain

36. What do footnotes do?

   A. Show the reader how ideas are organized

   B. Illustrate ideas that cannot clearly be stated in words

   C. Provide source information and peripheral information

   D. Provide nutrition facts about the contents of a package

37. Which of the following is a form of faulty reasoning?

   A. An overgeneralization

   B. A statement of opinion

   C. A documented statistic

   D. A verifiable piece of information

Read the following passage and answer questions 38-41.

Working mothers are required to perform a balancing act between their work and home lives every day or else everything will fall apart. Not only do they have mounds of work responsibilities, but also are expected to be the primary caregiver as well as the cook, cleaner, and organizer at home. Even though times have changed and more fathers are involved in parenting and home duties, the onus ultimately still falls on the working mother. Working mothers are shortchanged because they rarely get the chance to sit back and allow someone else to assume their responsibilities.

38. **What is the primary argument in the passage?**

A. Working mothers have it hard.

B. More mothers have entered the work force.

C. Fathers today are more willing to pitch in at home.

D. Working mothers cannot survive without the help of fathers.

39. **What assumption in this passage reflects negative stereotypical thinking?**

A. Fathers have jobs just like mothers do.

B. A lot of mothers today have full-time jobs.

C. Today's fathers are more involved at home.

D. Mothers cook, clean, and care for the children.

40. **The above argument is invalid because the author:**

A. suggests that working mothers choose to have such hectic lives.

B. uses derogatory and disrespectful language to describe fathers.

C. describes working mothers in a negative way that makes it seem as though they only look out for themselves.

D. professes an interest in all that working mothers do while simultaneously suggesting that fathers don't do enough.

41. **Re-read the following sentence from the passage:**

Working mothers are required to perform a balancing act between their work and home lives every day or else everything will fall apart.

What type of faulty reasoning does this sentence display?

A. Either/or fallacy

B. Circular reasoning

C. Bandwagon argument

D. False statement of cause and effect

42. **What is the best definition of the word *argument* in the context of reading and writing?**

A. An eloquent summary

B. An angry conversation

C. A persuasive point in a text

D. An object or direct object phrase

Study the infographic below and answer questions 43-44.

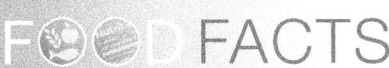

FOOD FACTS

Safe Food Handling: Four Simple Steps

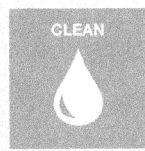 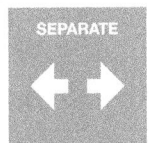  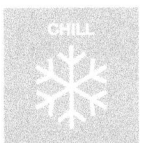

| CLEAN | SEPARATE | COOK | CHILL |

CLEAN
Wash hands and surfaces often

- Wash your hands with warm water and soap for at least 20 seconds before and after handling food and after using the bathroom, changing diapers, and handling pets.
- Wash your cutting boards, dishes, utensils, and counter tops with hot soapy water after preparing each food item.
- Consider using paper towels to clean up kitchen surfaces. If you use cloth towels, launder them often in the hot cycle.
- Rinse fresh fruits and vegetables under running tap water, including those with skins and rinds that are not eaten. Scrub firm produce with a clean produce brush.
- With canned goods, remember to clean lids before opening.

SEPARATE
Separate raw meats from other foods

- Separate raw meat, poultry, seafood, and eggs from other foods in your grocery shopping cart, grocery bags, and refrigerator.
- Use one cutting board for fresh produce and a separate one for raw meat, poultry, and seafood.
- Never place cooked food on a plate that previously held raw meat, poultry, seafood, or eggs unless the plate has been washed in hot, soapy water.
- Don't reuse marinades used on raw foods unless you bring them to a boil first.

COOK
Cook to the right temperature

- Color and texture are unreliable indicators of safety. Using a food thermometer is the only way to ensure the safety of meat, poultry, seafood, and egg products for all cooking methods. These foods must be cooked to a safe minimum internal temperature to destroy any harmful bacteria.
- Cook eggs until the yolk and white are firm. Only use recipes in which eggs are cooked or heated thoroughly.
- When cooking in a microwave oven, cover food, stir, and rotate for even cooking. If there is no turntable, rotate the dish by hand once or twice during cooking. Always allow standing time, which completes the cooking, before checking the internal temperature with a food thermometer.
- Bring sauces, soups and gravy to a boil when reheating.

CHILL
Refrigerate foods promptly

- Use an appliance thermometer to be sure the temperature is consistently 40° F or below and the freezer temperature is 0° F or below.
- Refrigerate or freeze meat, poultry, eggs, seafood, and other perishables within 2 hours of cooking or purchasing. Refrigerate within 1 hour if the temperature outside is above 90° F.
- Never thaw food at room temperature, such as on the counter top. There are three safe ways to defrost food: in the refrigerator, in cold water, and in the microwave. Food thawed in cold water or in the microwave should be cooked immediately.
- Always marinate food in the refrigerator.
- Divide large amounts of leftovers into shallow containers for quicker cooling in the refrigerator.

April 2017

For more information, contact the U.S. Food and Drug Administration, Center for Food Safety and Applied Nutrition's Food and Cosmetic Information Center at **1-888-SAFEFOOD** (toll free), Monday through Friday 10 AM to 4 PM ET (except Thursdays from 12:30 PM to 1:30 PM ET and Federal holidays). Or, visit the FDA website at **http://www.fda.gov/educationresourcelibrary**

Resource: The Food and Drug Administration

43. Which of the following is a sign that the infographic is credible?

A. The information is presented in an organized way.

B. The information comes from a government agency.

C. The information is colorful and engaging.

D. The information has the word "FACTS" written at the top.

44. What could a skeptical reader do to verify the facts on the infographic?

A. Interview one chef from a local restaurant about safe food handling

B. Contact the agencies whose phone numbers are listed at the bottom of the page

C. Check a tertiary source like Wikipedia to verify the information

D. Compare the info graphic's information about safe food handling to a cook's blog

45. Which sources are usually considered most trustworthy?

A. Primary sources

B. Secondary sources

C. Tertiary sources

D. Quaternary sources

46. A source is not credible if:

A. its publisher is government funded.

B. any of its sources are primary sources.

C. any of its sources are secondary sources.

D. its publisher is profiting from the information.

47. A(n) _____ may contain emotional arguments and still be considered credible because its purpose is to present an argument.

A. opinion article

B. scientific study

C. parenting guide

D. health textbook

48. Which type of evidence would not be considered credible to back up arguments in a persuasive text?

A. Logic   C. Scare tactics

B. Statistics   D. Firsthand accounts

49. A source is considered credible if readers can _____ it.

A. trust   C. analyze

B. publish   D. decipher

50. What type of source is an article about the latest Academy Award nominees by a Hollywood movie reviewer?

A. Primary   C. Tertiary

B. Secondary   D. None of the above

51. In literature, a genre is a:

A. moral.   C. category.

B. theme.   D. narrative.

52. When we discuss the _____ of a text, we are talking about how it is organized.

A. genre   C. structure

B. purpose   D. description

53. Narrative writing:

    A. tells a story.

    B. explains an idea.

    C. describes a process.

    D. makes an argument.

SECTION II. MATHEMATICS

You will have 54 minutes to complete 36 questions.

1. Jacob needs to get an 80% or higher on his language proficiency exam to earn school credit. If the exam has 120 questions, how many must he answer correctly?

   A. 100
   B. 96
   C. 80
   D. 106

2. Write 1.5 as a percent.

   A. 0.15%
   B. 1.5%
   C. 15%
   D. 150%

3. Harrison leaves the house driving at an average speed of 60 miles per hour on his way to work which is 40 miles away. After 20 miles, he gets stuck in a traffic jam for half an hour. After the jam, how fast does he need to drive if he wants to get to work in 15 minutes?

   A. 80 mph
   B. 60 mph
   C. 75 mph
   D. 65 mph

4. A tree has a circumference of 340 centimeters. Find the diameter to the nearest tenth of a centimeter. Use 3.14 for π.

   A. 27.1
   B. 54.1
   C. 81.4
   D. 108.3

5. Convert 6 meters to feet. (Note: 1 meter is equal to 3.28 feet.)

   A. 1.52 feet
   B. 1.72 feet
   C. 18.68 feet
   D. 19.68 feet

6. Siobhan walks 1.45 miles to school and then back home each day Monday through Friday. How many miles does she walk each week?

   A. 7.25
   B. 10.15
   C. 14.5
   D. 20.3

7. A box in the shape of a right rectangular prism has dimensions of 6 centimeters by 7 centimeters by 8 centimeters. What is the volume in cubic centimeters? (Note: V = length × width × height.)

   A. 280
   B. 336
   C. 560
   D. 672

8. Convert 9 pints to liters. (Note: 1 pint is equal to 0.473 liters.)

   A. 4.25 liters
   B. 4.50 liters
   C. 8.49 liters
   D. 9.54 liters

9. Benjamin buys $3\frac{1}{3}$, $2\frac{1}{2}$, and $1\frac{3}{4}$ of yards of fabric at a store. How many total yards did he purchase?

   A. $6\frac{5}{12}$
   B. $6\frac{5}{9}$
   C. $7\frac{7}{12}$
   D. $7\frac{7}{9}$

10. Julian earns a bonus at work worth 4.2% of his yearly salary. How much was Julian's bonus if his yearly salary is $65,000?

    A. $27,300
    B. $27.30
    C. $2,730
    D. $273.00

11. Solve the equation for the unknown.
    $$2(x-4) = 5(x + 2)$$

    A. −24
    B. −12
    C. −6
    D. −2

97

12. The box plot shows the number of students taking different busses to school. Which statement is true for the box plot?

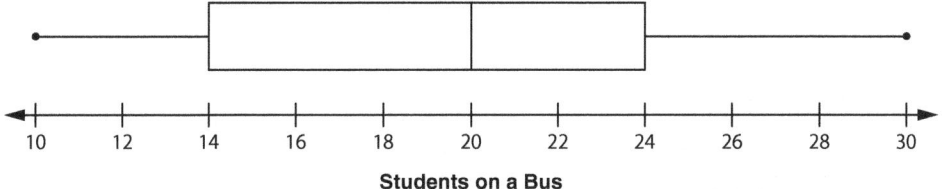

Students on a Bus

A. Half of the buses have 20 or fewer students.

B. Half of the buses have 24 or fewer students.

C. The difference between the maximum and minimum is 10 students.

D. The difference between the maximum and minimum is 14 students.

13. Select a histogram for the data below.

The data below show the number of cars that drove through an intersection on a Saturday.

1, 48, 60, 43, 41, 70, 75, 80, 101, 90, 121, 114, 99, 153, 205, 175, 222, 96, 201, 158, 141, 117, 74, 29

A.

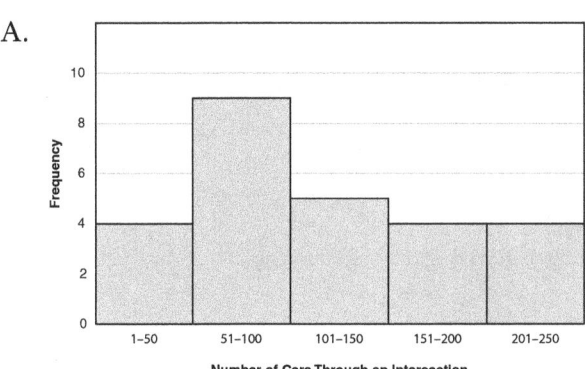

C.

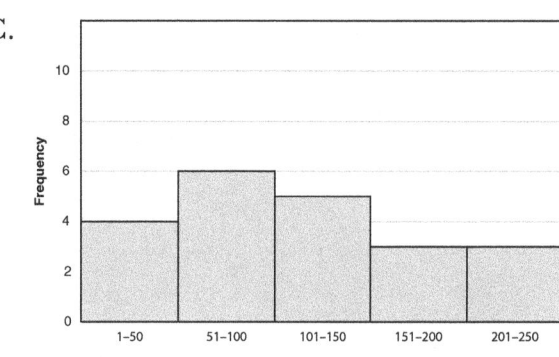

B.

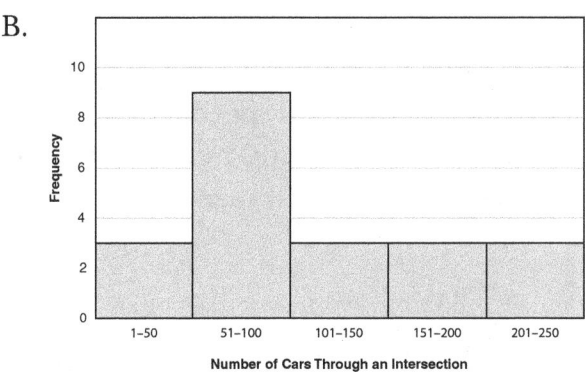

D.

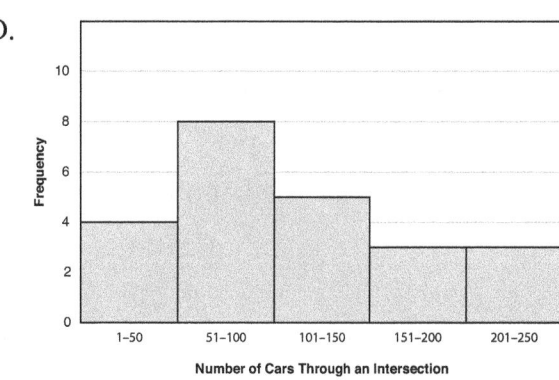

14. $3\frac{1}{4} \times 2\frac{2}{3}$

    A. $6\frac{1}{2}$ C. $8\frac{1}{2}$

    B. $6\frac{2}{3}$ D. $8\frac{2}{3}$

15. The original height of a plant is 1.75 inches. The plant grows an average of 1.08 inches each month for 6 months. What is the new height of the plant in inches?

    A. 7.13   C. 8.13

    B. 7.23   D. 8.23

16. If a waitress receives a $7.25 tip on top of a $40.28 bill, what percent did the customers tip her?

    A. 15.3%   C. 33%

    B. 8.2%   D. 18%

17. Solve for the value of y when $x = 2$.

    $y = (x^3 - 3) \times 2$

    A. 10   C. 12

    B. 6   D. 9

18. Solve the equation for the unknown.

    $-x - 15 = -17$

    A. −2   C. 1

    B. −1   D. 2

19. The number 22 is what percent of 54?

    A. 22%   C. 41%

    B. 29%   D. 76%

20. How many dogs are necessary to make a cat-to-dog ratio of 3:2 in an area with 1,425 cats?

    A. 285   C. 2,138

    B. 950   D. 2,375

21. Write $\frac{1}{5}$ as a percent.

    A. 15%   C. 25%

    B. 20%   D. 30%

22. A baker makes 5 dozen cupcakes and sells $\frac{5}{6}$ of them for $2 each. How much money did she make?

    A. $60   C. $120

    B. $50   D. $100

23. Write 12.5% as a fraction.

    A. $\frac{1}{12}$ C. $\frac{1}{8}$

    B. $\frac{1}{9}$ D. $\frac{1}{7}$

24. Find the difference.

    $\frac{15}{16} - \frac{3}{8}$

    A. $\frac{3}{4}$ C. $\frac{7}{8}$

    B. $\frac{9}{16}$ D. $\frac{1}{2}$

25. If a truck's initial speed is 60 mph and its final speed is 100 mph, what is its percent change in speed?

    A. 17%   C. 40%

    B. 33%   D. 67%

26. A start up company with 30 employees grows to 70 employees in 6 months. If it continues to grow at the same rate, what is the employee increase after one year?

    A. $2\frac{2}{3}$ C. 2

    B. $1\frac{2}{3}$ D. $2\frac{1}{3}$

27. The table shows the speed in miles per hour of different roller coasters at an amusement park. Select the correct line graph for this data.

Amusement Park Roller Coasters	1	2	3	4	5	6	7	8
Speed (miles per hour)	120	105	75	100	60	85	110	90

A.

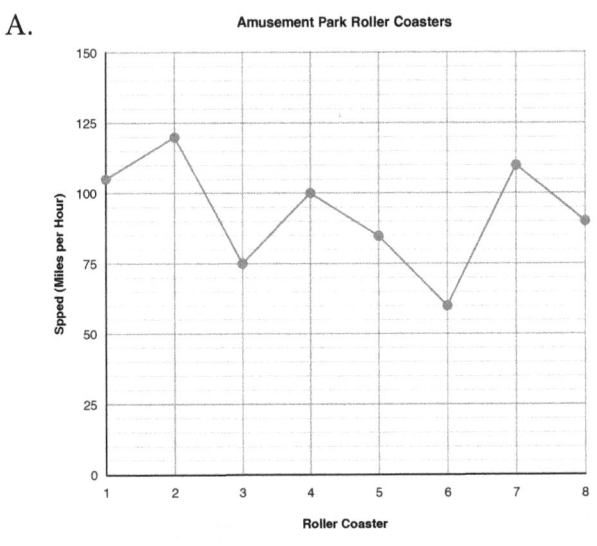

C.

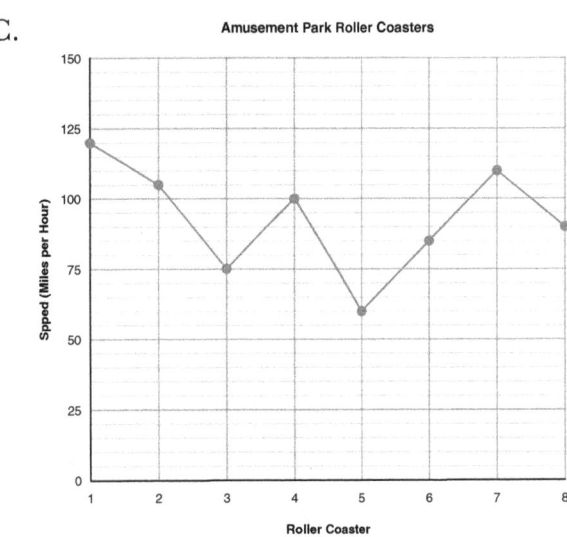

B.

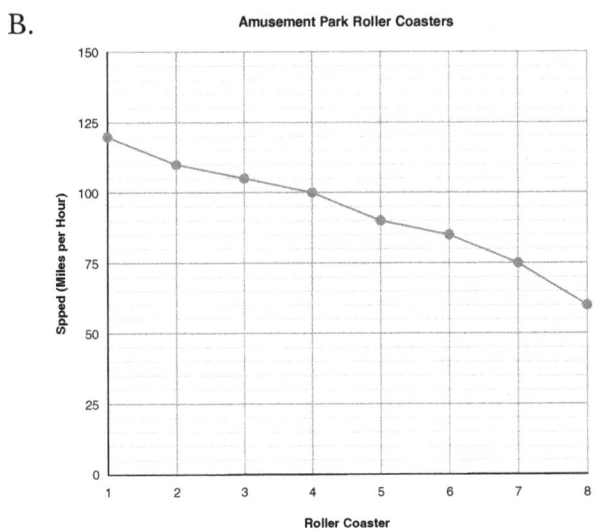

D.

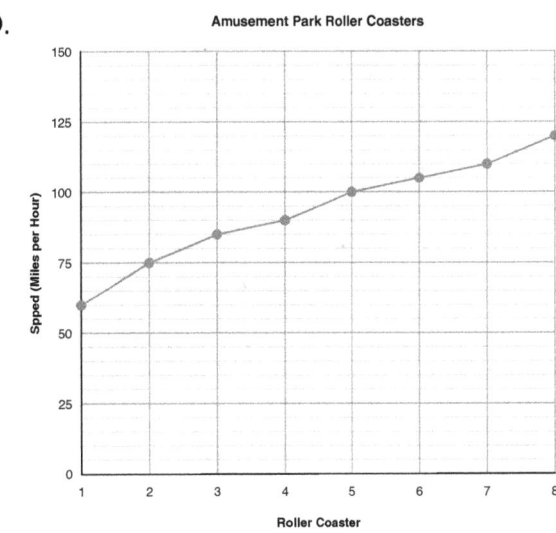

28. The circle graph shows the number of votes for each candidate. How many votes were cast for candidate D if there were 25,000 voters?

Votes for Candidate

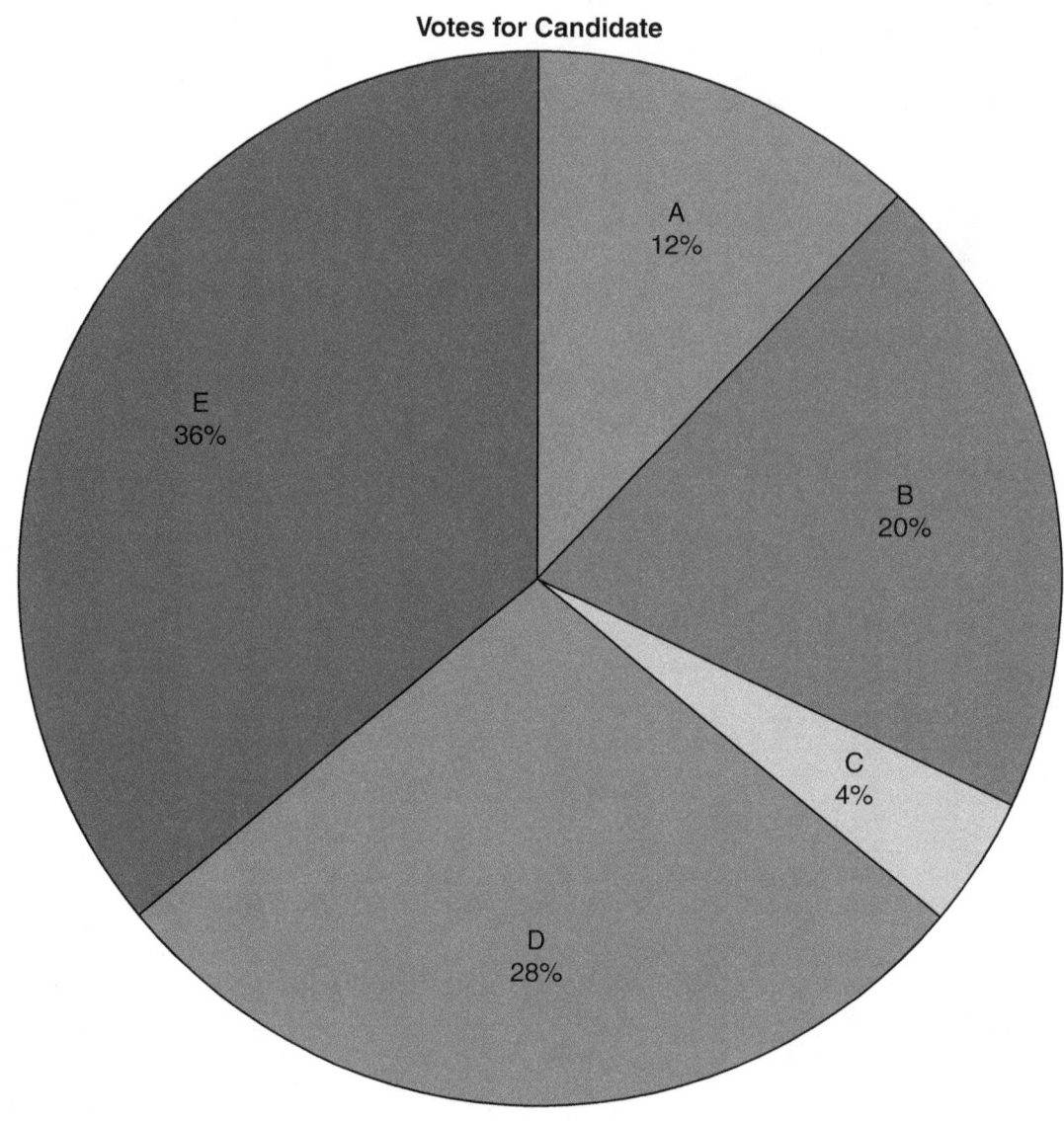

A. 3,000 votes

B. 5,000 votes

C. 7,000 votes

D. D.9,000 votes

29. The bar chart shows the number of boys and girls who participate in sports. What is the greatest difference between numbers of participants in any year?

Sports Participants

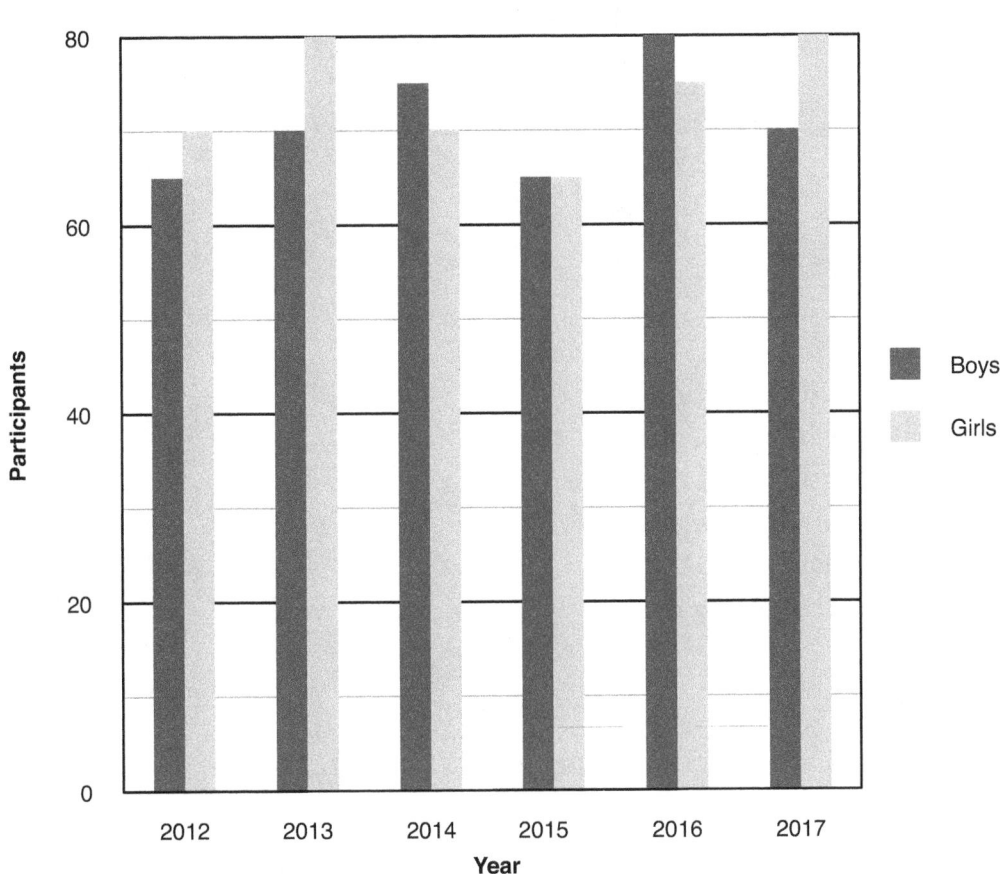

A. 0

C. 10

B. 5

D. 15

30. A builder buys 3 boxes of different sized screws, each containing 450 screws. If he uses $\frac{1}{3}$ of one box, $\frac{1}{6}$ of another, and $\frac{3}{5}$ of the biggest sized screw, how many total screws does he have left?

A. 795

C. 1,350

B. 300

D. 855

31. Grandma Sarah baked cookies for her grandchildren. If Sarah's eldest grandchild ate 1/3 of the cookies and she made 120 cookies total, how many cookies remain for the other grandchildren?

A. 80

C. 60

B. 100

D. 75

32. Solve for x when $(\sqrt{4})x = 6^2$

A. 3

C. 9

B. 18

D. 24

33. Perform the operation.

$(-2x^2 + 8x) + (3x^3 - 4x^2 + 1)$

A. $3x^3 - 6x^2 + 8x + 1$

B. $3x^3 - 2x^2 + 8x + 1$

C. $3x^3 + 6x^2 + 8x + 1$

D. $3x^3 + 2x^2 + 8x + 1$

34. $1\frac{5}{6} \div 1\frac{1}{3}$

A. $1\frac{5}{18}$ C. $2\frac{4}{9}$

B. $1\frac{3}{8}$ D. $3\frac{1}{6}$

35. A pharmacist needs to fill a prescription of 10 grams (g) of medicine in the form of pills. If the pills are designed to be 100 milligrams (mg) of medicine each, how many pills does the pharmacist need to fill the prescription? (Note: 1g is equal to 1,000mg.)

A. 1,000 C. 10

B. 100 D. 1

36. A patient has a fever of 105°C. What is this value in Fahrenheit? (Note: $°F = \frac{9}{5}°C + 32$).

A. 137 C. 189

B. 157 D. 221

SECTION III. SCIENCE

You have 63 minutes to complete 53 questions.

1. The skin and linings of internal organs are examples of what type of tissue?

   A. Connective
   C. Muscle
   B. Epithelial
   D. Neural

2. Which type of tissue coordinates and controls many body activities?

   A. Connective
   C. Muscle
   B. Epithelial
   D. Neural

3. What substances transported in blood does the liver excrete as bile?

   A. Gases
   C. Nutrients
   B. Hormones
   D. Wastes

4. What is the purpose of the superior vena cava?

   A. Flow blood into the pulmonary artery

   B. Facilitate blood drainage into the right ventricle

   C. Carries deoxygenated blood from the upper half of the body to the right atrium

   D. Saturate the body tissues with a large volume of blood

5. The negative-feedback mechanism that regulates the level of glucose in a person's blood is an example of what type of hormone secretion regulation?

   A. Hormone regulation

   B. Nervous system regulation

   C. Blood levels of chemical regulation

   D. Intercellular ion concentration regulation

6. Which chemical signal would respond to the redness caused by an infected wound?

   A. Autocrines

   B. Neuromodulators

   C. Paracrines

   D. Pheromones

7. Which of the following is one of the primary functions of the endocrine system?

   A. Blood glucose control

   B. Digestive system control

   C. Nervous system regulation

   D. Negative feedback initiation

8. What is the primary function of the oral cavity?

   A. Diffusion

   B. Digestion

   C. Lubrication

   D. Mastication

9. Where are the sublingual salivary glands located?

   A. Near the ears

   B. Below the jaw

   C. Under the tongue

   D. Beside the sinuses

10. Which of the following is one of the primary functions of the large intestine?

   A. To kill bacteria

   B. To recycle water

   C. To store excess fats

   D. To reduce the amount of waste

11. Where in the nail bed is the lunula found?

   A. Area of white space

   B. Thick overhang layer

   C. Region of epidermal cells

   D. Collection of keratinized cells

12. How many epidermal layers make up the face?

   A. 3   C. 5
   B. 4   D. 6

13. What region of the skin is targeted for correction of saggy, thin skin?

   A. Dermal layer

   B. Hypodermis layer

   C. Stratum corneum

   D. Stratum spinosum

14. Which heart layer is composed primarily of cardiac muscle?

   A. Myocardium

   B. Pericardium

   C. Septum

   D. Sternum

15. Which of the following has already occured once the third line of cellular defense has begun?

   A. The B cells flagged the pathogen.

   B. Histamines blocked the pathogen.

   C. The patrolling macrophages missed the pathogen.

   D. Killer T cells were unable to destroy the pathogen.

16. Which of the following describes the characteristic that all muscles recoil after stretching?

   A. elastic   C. excitable

   B. relaxing   D. contractile

17. Which of the following is a muscle cell?

   A. Fascicle   C. Muscle fiber

   B. Sarcomere   D. Actin myofilament

18. When a flexor muscles contracts, an extension muscle _____.

   A. elongates   C. recoils

   B. pivots   D. shortens

19. What lobe helps a person interpret information received from the retinas of the eyes?

   A. Frontal   C. Parietal

   B. Occipital   D. Temporal

20. The hypothalamus works directly with the _____ to control the body using hormones.

   A. amygdala

   B. hippocampus

   C. pituitary gland

   D. skeletal muscle

21. **Which neuroglia produces myelin sheaths?**

    A. Satellite cells

    B. Schwann cells

    C. Microglial cells

    D. Ependymal cells

22. **What increases electric signal transmission through a neuron?**

    A. Axon terminal

    B. Myelin sheath

    C. Resting potential

    D. Synaptic transmission

23. **Which of the following is generally true regarding human newborns?**

    A. Newborns require a large amount of parental care.

    B. Newborns enter the first stages of puberty within a few weeks of birth.

    C. Newborns are capable of sexually reproducing within a few months of birth.

    D. Newborns are able to visually track objects with their eyes moments after delivery.

24. **What changes occur in a female body after fertilization takes place?**

    A. Puberty begins.

    B. Hormonal changes signal pregnancy.

    C. Menstruation stops due to menopause.

    D. Menstruation occurs within a few weeks.

25. **Which organ uses hairs to filter out particles that try to enter the lungs?**

    A. Alveoli   C. Larynx

    B. Bronchus   D. Nose

26. **Which describes pulmonary ventilation?**

    A. Air movement into and out of the lungs

    B. Transportation of blood into circulation

    C. Gas exchange between blood and lungs

    D. Diffusion of blood to cells in body tissues

27. **What happens when the diaphragm moves down?**

    A. The ribs move inward.

    B. A person is able to exhale.

    C. Air is drawn into the lungs.

    D. Alveolar surface area decreases.

28. **What does an X-ray reveal when imaging a bone within the lower extremities?**

    A. Skull   C. Rib cage

    B. Hyoid   D. Metatarsals

29. **How many bones make up the pectoral girdle?**

    A. 4   C. 60

    B. 6   D. 80

30. **Which of the following is a short bone?**

    A. Carpal   C. Scapula

    B. Patella   D. Tibia

31. **Which is a characteristic of the bladder?**
    A. Stores urine
    B. Filters blood
    C. Shaped like a bean
    D. Reddish-brown in color

32. **Which function is the glomerulus responsible for?**
    A. Filtering
    B. Excretion
    C. Circulating
    D. Reabsorption

33. **Which bonds are used to join water molecules together?**
    A. Covalent
    B. Hydrogen
    C. Ionic
    D. Peptide

34. **Which of the following is produced during the citric acid cycle?**
    A. Electrons
    B. NADH
    C. Pyruvate
    D. Cellulose

35. **How many molecules of ATP are produced after glycolysis?**
    A. 2
    B. 9
    C. 12
    D. 32

36. **Why is glycolysis a catabolic pathway?**
    A. Electrons are transferred from one molecule to another.
    B. Energy is released as glucose splits into pyruvate molecules.
    C. Several different types of molecules are formed as products.
    D. Different biomolecules used during this process are reduced.

37. **What cellular process do autotrophs rely on to obtain energy?**
    A. Carbon fixation
    B. Cell respiration
    C. Photosynthesis
    D. Gluconeogenesis

38. **Which cell part is associated with both animal and plant cells?**
    A. Cell wall
    B. Chloroplast
    C. Large vacuole
    D. Endoplasmic reticulum

39. **How many rounds of cell division occur during meiosis?**
    A. 1
    B. 2
    C. 3
    D. 4

40. **If someone needs ATP desperately and has run out of oxygen, what could help?**
    A. Meiosis
    B. Calvin cycle
    C. Fermentation
    D. Electron transport chain

41. **A child falls down and punctures his skin. What biological process must occur to repair the damaged skin?**
    A. Glycolysis
    B. Cell Respiration
    C. Gluconeogenesis
    D. Cell Reproduction

42. In DNA replication, a DNA strand is separated, and a

    A. complementary strand attaches.

    B. complementary strand is assembled.

    C. complementary strand replicates itself.

    D. complementary strand forms a double helix.

43. An offspring receives _____ allele(s) for a particular trait from each parent.

    A. 1   C. 3

    B. 2   D. 4

44. Once RNA polymerase reaches a stop codon on the DNA molecule, the enzyme detaches from the DNA and releases the RNA molecule

    A. into the cell for the next stage.

    B. into the cytoplasm for translation.

    C. into the nucleus for the next stage.

    D. into the cytoplasm for transcription.

45. The replication of DNA ends with a twisted strand called a _____.

    A. base pair

    B. nucleic acid

    C. double helix

    D. single strand

46. Why is the metric system used in science?

    A. The base units are used interchangeably.

    B. It is easy to remember how the system works.

    C. The units are expressed as a base of a hundred.

    D. It is a universally accepted way to report values.

47. Which part of the scientific method requires a researcher to create variables?

    A. Writing a procedure

    B. Testing a hypothesis

    C. Drafting a conclusion

    D. Formulating a hypothesis

48. The combustion reaction for butane (C_4H_{10}), the fuel inside lighters, is shown below. What coefficient must be added to oxygen (O_2) to balance this equation?

    $2C_4H_{10} + \underline{\quad}O_2 \rightarrow 8CO_2 + 10H_2O$

    A. 8   C. 13

    B. 9   D. 18

49. Atom X has an atomic number of 10 and a mass of 20 amu. Atom Y has 10 protons and 12 neutrons. Which of the following describes the relationship between these atoms?

    A. They are different elements.

    B. They are isotopes of the same element.

    C. They have the same atomic number and the same atomic mass.

    D. They have different atomic numbers and different atomic masses.

50. An atom contains 15 protons, 16 neutrons, and 18 electrons. What element is it? (refer to the periodic table of elements)

A. Argon

B. Phosphorus

C. Selenium

D. Sulfur

51. Why are water molecules attracted to themselves?

A. As a result of the polar configuration

B. As a result of the physical configuration

C. As a result of the intensive configuration

D. As a result of the extensive configuration

52. What is the goal of osmosis?

A. The water will equalize on both side of the semipermeable membrane.

B. The concentration of solutes will diffuse through the semipermeable membrane.

C. The concentration of free water molecules will equalize on both sides of the membrane

D. The solute particles will flow from an area of high concentration to an area of lower concentration.

53. The amount of heat that has been removed from the substance allows the particles to draw closer together, and the material changes from a liquid to a solid. Which of the following is being described?

A. Condensation

B. Deposition

C. Freezing

D. Sublimation

SECTION IV. ENGLISH AND LANGUAGE USAGE

You have 28 minutes to complete 28 questions.

1. **Which of the following is correct?**

    A. senate

    B. congress

    C. White House

    D. Supreme court

2. **Which of the following sentences is correct?**

    A. I asked Scott, How was your day?

    B. Scott said, it was awesome.

    C. He claimed, "My history presentation was great!"

    D. I said, That's wonderful!

3. **What is the correct plural of *morning*?**

    A. Morning   C. Morninges

    B. Mornings   D. Morningies

4. **How many nouns in the following sentence have incorrect capitalization?**

    The Patel Family moved to the United States, and now they live in the Boston Area.

    A. 0   C. 2

    B. 1   D. 3

5. **Which of the following pronouns correctly completes this sentence?**

    Mrs. Sato, _____ lives down the street, is 99 years old.

    A. she   C. which

    B. who   D. whom

6. **Which word in the following sentence is an adjective?**

    After they signed the mortgage on their first house, they went out to celebrate.

    A. they   C. mortgage

    B. signed   D. first

7. **Identify the conjunction in the following sentence.**

    He is sick, yet he came to work.

    A. is   C. came

    B. yet   D. to

8. **Which of the following correctly describes both of these verbs: "offered" and "advised"?**

    When a buyer <u>offered</u> 5% below our asking price, our realtor <u>advised</u> us to accept the offer.

    A. Helping verbs

    B. Past tense verbs

    C. Present tense verbs

    D. Progressive tense verbs

9. **Which of the following verbs correctly completes this sentence?**

    Do you think the automobile or the personal computer _____ changed our lives more?

    A. have   C. has

    B. haves   D. his

10. **Which of the following verbs has the word "she" as its subject in this sentence?**

After we add the flour, <u>she</u> wants us to stir the mixture really well.

A. add   C. us

B. wants   D. stir

11. **Which of the following verbs correctly completes this sentence?**

Where ____ everyone? What ____ they doing?

A. is, is   C. are, is

B. is, are   D. are, are

12. **Fill in the blank with the correct coordinating conjunction.**

My friend and I went to dinner, _____ we both ordered pasta.

A. so   C. but

B. or   D. and

13. **Identify the dependent clause in the following sentence.**

While her kids swam in the pool, Nicole read a book.

A. While her kids swam in the pool

B. Nicole read a book

C. Swam in the pool

D. While her kids

14. **Which of the following uses a conjunction to combine the sentences below so the focus is on Tony preparing for his job interview?**

Tony prepared well for his job interview. Tony ended up getting an offer.

A. Tony ended up getting an offer; he prepared for his job interview.

B. Tony prepared well for his job interview, he ended up getting an offer.

C. Tony prepared well for his job interview and he ended up getting an offer.

D. Tony ended up getting an offer because he prepared for his job interview.

15. **Which sentence combines all this information using a parallel structure?**

Dental care requires brushing. You should also floss. Rinse with a fluoride wash.

A. Dental care requires to brush, floss, and rinsing.

B. Dental care requires brushing, to floss, and rinse.

C. Dental care requires brushing, flossing, and rinse.

D. Dental care requires brushing, flossing, and rinsing.

16. Which of the following options correctly fixes the fragment below?

During the movie.

A. During the movie I spilled my popcorn.

B. During the movie, I spilled my popcorn.

C. During the movie. I spilled my popcorn.

D. During the movie, and I spilled my popcorn.

17. Which of the following sentences uses the MOST informal language?

A. I talk to him sporadically.

B. I need to get dressed.

C. You'll be okay.

D. The air outside is chilly.

18. Which of the following sentences uses the MOST formal language?

A. Please send me a timely response.

B. Give me a response.

C. Please tell me.

D. Respond.

19. Which of the following words in this sentence has more than one meaning?

Officials were worried that the bad weather would hamper their search efforts.

A. Officials   C. Weather

B. Worried   D. Hamper

20. Which of the following is the meaning of "buckle" as used in this sentence?

Cassandra was about to buckle from all the pressures of her new job.

A. To attack

B. To fasten together

C. To collapse or bend

D. To start to work hard

21. Which of the following context clues correctly helps you define the word "cabinet" in this sentence?

The cabinet advised the young president on what to do about the hostage situation.

A. "advised"   C. "hostage"

B. "young"   D. "situation"

22. Which of the following is the meaning of "morose" as used in this sentence?

After his wife's death, the man became morose and would not talk to anyone.

A. Mute   C. Isolated

B. Glum   D. Embarrassed

23. Which of the following context clues correctly helps you define the word "loquacious" in this sentence?

The loquacious politician droned on during his speech about tax reform.

A. "politician"   C. "about "

B. "droned on"   D. "tax reform"

24. *Irascible* most nearly means

A. easily angered.

B. easily swayed.

C. easily amused.

D. easily embarrassed.

25. **Which of the following is the meaning of "rejuvenate" as used in this sentence?**

Spending the day getting pampered at a spa will <u>rejuvenate</u> anyone.

A. Make someone feel sleepy

B. Make someone feel relaxed

C. Make someone feel young again

D. Make someone feel appreciative

26. **A kleptomaniac is someone who**

A. steals.

B. overeats.

C. lights fires.

D. pretends to be sick.

27. **Which of the following suffixes means "one who loves"?**

A. -or

B. -er

C. -ist

D. -phile

28. **Which of the following root words means "color"?**

A. *vid*

B. *chron*

C. *chrom*

D. *therm*

TEAS Practice Exam 3
Answer Key with Explanatory Answers

Section I. Reading

1. D. This narrative paragraph about a fed-up young mother suggests its main idea rather than stating it outright. There is no topic sentence. **Skill: Main Ideas, Topic Sentences, and Supporting Details.**

2. C. The best statement of an implied main idea stays true to the words and ideas the author actually shares. In this case, the central idea is Faith's frustration with other people's reminiscences. **Skill: Main Ideas, Topic Sentences, and Supporting Details.**

3. D. The topic of this paragraph the benefits of dark chocolate. **Skill: Main Ideas, Topic Sentences, and Supporting Details.**

4. B. The second sentence of this paragraph leads the reader toward the main idea, which is that dark chocolate has health benefits. **Skill: Main Ideas, Topic Sentences, and Supporting Details.**

5. D. A popular recipe using dark chocolate as its main ingredient would be an off-topic sentence since it is not related to the main idea of the health benefits of dark chocolate. **Skill: Main Ideas, Topic Sentences, and Supporting Details.**

6. C. The description of the paragraph is not valid because the author of the paragraph ends with a warning to readers about its high caloric content. **Skill: Main Ideas, Topic Sentences, and Supporting Details.**

7. A. This statistic would be off-topic information in this paragraph because it is about all chocolate not the health benefits of dark chocolate. **Skill: Main Ideas, Topic Sentences, and Supporting Details.**

8. B. Even though the detail about Max setting up the picnic came at the end, it was the event that happened first since he had to have set up before Cynthia came to the park because it was there before they arrived. **Skill: Summarizing Text and Using Text Features.**

9. A. The word clues "had set up" indicates that Max set up the picnic earlier so that it would be a surprise for Cynthia when they got to the clearing. **Skill: Summarizing Text and Using Text Features.**

10. D. Even though the word "beginning" seems like a sequence word indicating something that comes first, in the context of the passage it means they "started to" get thirsty. The other words are sequence words, which indicate the order of events. **Skill: Summarizing Text and Using Text Features.**

11. C. This paragraph does not fully explain the connection between the opening point and the evidence in the quotation. **Skill: The Writing Process.**

12. D. The sentence about comparing waves to trees shows how the metaphor works in the poem. This completes the point begun in the first three sentences of the paragraph. **Skill: The Writing Process.**

13. B. Mind mapping is a brainstorming and organizational tool to help arrange associated ideas into a hierarchy. **Skill: The Writing Process.**

14. D. Revising is not just fixing mechanical errors; it involves making major changes to the content and structure of a draft. **Skill: The Writing Process.**

15. A. Citations are notes within a text about where the author got information. They are a vital part of research writing. **Skill: The Writing Process.**

16. D. Drafting is about getting ideas down on paper. You can reread later to fix awkward sentences and errors. **Skill: The Writing Process.**

17. B. The author needs more precise word choice in Sentence 1. A "bad" commercial could have poor acting or be unconvincing; in this case, the author is implying that the commercial is harmful to society. **Skill: Essay Revision and Transitions.**

18. A. The author's point is not necessarily that the TV commercial she saw should be banned. Rather, she is trying to convince women to share her outrage about the way society pressures them to look. **Skill: Essay Revision and Transitions.**

19. C. The thesis suggests that women should base their self-esteem on their accomplishments, but the body paragraphs mainly defend the point that the media presents unrealistic images of beauty. **Skill: Essay Revision and Transitions.**

20. A. The author does not actually defend the point that women should base their self-esteem on their accomplishments. Rather, the body paragraphs focus on the idea that the media's image of beauty is false. **Skill: Essay Revision and Transitions.**

21. B. The two body paragraphs are not strongly differentiated from each other. **Skill: Essay Revision and Transitions.**

22. D. Examples of women who deliberately minimize the time they spend on looking good do not belong in a paragraph claiming that most women spend too much time and money on beauty. **Skill: Essay Revision and Transitions.**

23. C. A transition word like *personally* at the beginning of Sentence 3 could signal that the writer is shifting from a description of a television commercial to her own opinion. **Skill: Essay Revision and Transitions.**

24. B. Academic essays should not use contractions. Note that this essay focuses specifically on pressures women face to look beautiful. In this case, the language does not need to be inclusive of both genders because that would change the meaning. **Skill: Essay Revision and Transitions.**

25. B. Word choice, or diction, is the reader's most important tool in determining tone. **Skill: Tone, Mood, and Transition Words.**

26. C. Mood is the feeling a text creates in a reader; tone is the author's attitude toward the subject. **Skill: Tone, Mood, and Transition Words.**

27. D. Tone is the author's apparent attitude toward the subject of a text. It is distinguished from mood, which is the reader's emotional response. **Skill: Tone, Mood, and Transition Words.**

28. A. Although the author of this passage seems to lean toward the negative impact of technology and youth, the passage does not actually make a clear argument. It only relays the survey results and words from an expert. **Skill: Understanding Author's Purpose, Point of View, and Rhetorical Strategies.**

29. A. The author of the passage is likely concerned with the negative impact technology is having on our youth since he/she only presents the cons of technology. **Skill: Understanding Author's Purpose, Point of View, and Rhetorical Strategies.**

30. B. Rhetorical strategies are techniques an author uses to develop a main idea. An effective way to do this is to appeal to the readers' reason by relying on factual information. The most effective reason is the one about a recent screen time study. It shows that technology use has risen since it's available in so many forms. This is a fact that can be proven. **Skill: Understanding Author's Purpose, Point of View, and Rhetorical Strategies.**

31. A. The passage first reports on the results of a survey about technology use and young people. Greensburg's comments explain the effects this technology is having on young people. **Skill: Understanding Author's Purpose, Point of View, and Rhetorical Strategies.**

32. D. Narrative works like science fiction novels are usually meant to entertain. **Skill: Understanding the Author's Purpose, Point of View, and Rhetorical Strategies.**

33. C. The bottom row shows the range of lengths likely for a 6.5-month-old baby. The rightmost column shows the 97th percentile value for each age group. **Skill: Evaluating and Integrating Data.**

34. C. Candice is unusually tall for her age, so her length falls outside the values included in the chart. It is not impossible for her to be this tall; her height is above the 97th percentile. **Skill: Evaluating and Integrating Data.**

35. C. An article that takes a moral position is meant to persuade. **Skill: Understanding the Author's Purpose, Point of View, and Rhetorical Strategies.**

36. C. Footnotes may provide information about source materials or give the reader interesting information that is not essential to the main point. **Skill: Evaluating and Integrating Data.**

37. A. An overgeneralization is a broad claim based on too little evidence, so this would be an example of faulty reasoning. **Skill: Facts, Opinions, and Evaluating an Argument.**

38. A. This passage argues that working mothers have it hard. **Skill: Facts, Opinions, and Evaluating an Argument.**

39. D. The writer of this passage makes the assumption that mothers cook, clean, and care for the children. **Skill: Facts, Opinions, and Evaluating an Argument.**

40. D. The author of the passage uses the phrase "the onus ultimately still falls on the working mother." This implies that fathers do not do enough to help out. **Skill: Facts, Opinions, and Evaluating an Argument.**

41. A. This statement takes a complex issue and presents it as if only two possible options are in play. This is an either/or fallacy. **Skill: Facts, Opinions, and Evaluating an Argument.**

42. C. In the context of reading and writing, an argument is a statement meant to prove a point, not a heated disagreement. **Skill: Facts Opinions and Evaluating an Argument.**

43. B. The information comes a government agency called the FDA, and government sources are credible. **Skill: Understanding Primary Sources, Making Inferences, and Drawing Conclusions.**

44. B. One way to verify facts is to call all the numbers of the government agencies listed at the bottom of the page for more information. **Skill: Understanding Primary Sources, Making Inferences, and Drawing Conclusions.**

45. A. The authors of primary sources witnessed the original creation or discovery of the information they present. For this reason, they are considered the most trustworthy. **Skill: Understanding Primary Sources Making Inferences and Drawing Conclusions.**

46. D. A text is highly unlikely to be credible if its publisher is an organization that stands to benefit if people believe the information it contains. **Skill: Understanding Primary Sources, Making Inferences, and Drawing Conclusions.**

47. A. An opinion argument may include emotional language and still be credible as long as it is not manipulative. **Skill: Understanding Primary Sources, Making Inferences, and Drawing Conclusions.**

48. C. Emotional arguments may reasonably appear in a persuasive text, but not if they use manipulative strategies like scare tactics. **Skill: Understanding Primary Sources, Making Inferences, and Drawing Conclusions.**

49. A. The word *credible* means "trustworthy." **Skill: Understanding Primary Sources, Making Inferences, and Drawing Conclusions.**

50. **B.** An article that presents a review, or one person's opinion, of a work of literature or movie is a secondary source. **Skill: Understanding Primary Sources, Making Inferences, and Drawing Conclusions.**

51. **C.** The word *genre* is synonym of *category*. We use the word *genre* to discuss categories of literature. **Skill: Types of Passages, Text Structures, Genre and Theme.**

52. **C.** A genre is a category of a text, and the purpose it what it is meant to do. The structure is how it is organized. **Skill: Types of Passages, Text Structures, Genre and Theme.**

53. **A.** Narrative writing may be fiction or nonfiction as long as it tells a story. **Skill: Types of Passages, Text Structures, Genre and Theme.**

Section II. Mathematics

1. **B.** Jacob needs to get 96 questions correct on the exam because 80% or $0.80 \times 120 = 96$. **Skill: Ratios, Proportions, and Percentages.**

2. **D.** The correct answer is 150% because 1.5 as a percent is $1.5 \times 100 = 150\%$. **Skill: Decimals and Fractions.**

3. **A.** Harrison needs to drive 80 miles per hour to make it to work in 15 minutes because he has 20 miles to go and (20 miles ÷ 15 minutes) × 60 minutes in an hour = 80 mph. **Skill: Solving Real World Mathematical Problems.**

4. **D.** The correct solution is 108.3 because $C = \pi d; 340 = 3.14d; d \approx 108.3$ centimeters. **Skill: Circles.**

5. **D.** The correct solution is 19.68 feet. $6 \text{ m} \times \frac{3.28 \text{ ft}}{1 \text{ m}} = 19.68 \text{ ft}$. **Skill: Standards of Measure.**

6. **C.** The correct solution is 14.5 because $1.45(10) = 14.5$ miles. **Skill: Solving Real World Mathematical Problems.**

7. **B.** The correct solution is 336. Substitute the values into the formula and simplify using the order of operations, $V = lwh = 6(7)(8)$ cubic centimeters. **Skill: Similarity, Right Triangles, and Trigonometry.**

8. **A.** The correct solution is 4.25 liters. $9 \text{ pt} \times \frac{1 \text{ qt}}{2 \text{ pt}} \times \frac{1 \text{ L}}{1.06 \text{ qt}} = \frac{9}{2.12} = 4.25 \text{ L}$. **Skill: Standards of Measure.**

9. **C.** The correct solution is $7\frac{7}{12}$ because $3\frac{1}{3} + 2\frac{1}{2} + 1\frac{3}{4} = 3\frac{4}{12} + 2\frac{6}{12} + 1\frac{9}{12} = 6\frac{19}{12} = 7\frac{7}{12}$ yards of fabric. **Skill: Solving Real World Mathematical Problems.**

10. **C.** Julian earned a bonus worth $2,730 because 4.2% is equivalent to 0.042. Multiplying the value by the salary shows $65,000 \times 0.042 = \$2,730$. **Skill: Ratios, Proportions, and Percentages.**

11. C. The correct solution is −6.

$2x-8 = 5x + 10$	Apply the distributive property.
$-3x-8 = 10$	Subtract $5x$ from both sides of the equation.
$-3x = 18$	Add 8 to both sides of the equation.
$x = -6$	Divide both sides of the equation by −3.

Skill: Equations with One Variable.

12. A. The correct solution is half of the buses have 20 or fewer students. The median value is 20, and half of the buses have fewer than the median value. **Skill: Interpreting Categorical and Quantitative Data.**

13. D. The correct solution is D. Each bin contains 50 cars, and the frequencies are 4, 8, 5, 3, and 3. **Skill: Interpreting Categorical and Quantitative Data.**

14. D. The correct solution is $8\frac{2}{3}$ because $\frac{13}{4} \times \frac{8}{3} = \frac{104}{12} = 8\frac{8}{12} = 8\frac{2}{3}$. **Skill: Multiplication and Division of Fractions.**

15. D. The correct solution is 8.23 because $1.75 + 1.08(6) = 1.75 + 6.48 = 8.23$ inches. **Skill: Solving Real World Mathematical Problems.**

16. D. The waitress received an 18% customer service tip because $\frac{\$7.25}{\$40.28} = \frac{X}{100}$ and $x = 0.18$ or 18%. **Skill: Ratios, Proportions, and Percentages.**

17. A. The correct solution is 10 because $x^3 = 8 - 3 = 5 \times 2 = 10$. **Skill: Equations with One Variable.**

18. D. The correct solution is 2.

$-x = -2$	Add 15 to both sides of the equation.
$x = 2$	Divide both sides of the equation by −1.

Skill: Equations with One Variable.

19. C. The fraction $\frac{22}{54}$ is 41%, meaning 22 is 41% of 54. **Skill: Ratios, Proportions, and Percentages.**

20. B. The correct answer is B. Set up the proportion of dogs to cats (or vice versa):

$$\frac{2}{3} = \frac{?}{1,425}$$

Since $1,425 \div 3 = 475$, the number of dogs is the product of 2 and 475, or 950. **Skill: Ratios, Proportions, and Percentages.**

21. B. The correct answer is 20% because $\frac{1}{5}$ as a percent is $0.2 \times 100 = 20\%$. **Skill: Decimals and Fractions**

22. D. The baker made $100 selling the cupcakes because she made 60 cupcakes altogether and sold 50 of them at $2 each. **Skill: Multiplication and Division of Fractions.**

23. **C.** The correct answer is $\frac{1}{8}$ because 12.5% as a fraction is $\frac{12.5}{100} = \frac{125}{1000} = \frac{1}{8}$. **Skill: Decimals and Fractions.**

24. **B.** The correct answer is $\frac{9}{16}$ because $\frac{15}{16} - \frac{3}{8} = \frac{15}{16} - \frac{6}{16} = \frac{9}{16}$. **Skill: Addition and Subtraction of Fractions.**

25. **D.** The truck has a 67% change in speed. The truck's change in speed is the difference between its final and initial speed: in this case, 100 mph − 60 mph = 40 mph. To find the percent change, divide 40 mph by the initial speed (60 mph) and then multiply by 100%.

$$\frac{40 \text{ mph}}{60 \text{ mph}} \times 100\% = 0.67 \times 100\% = 67\%$$

Skill: Ratios, Proportions, and Percentages.

26. **A.** The company increases by 40 employees within 6 months, and would likely have an additional 80 employees within the year. $\frac{80}{30} = 2\frac{2}{3}$ increase in employees. **Skill: Multiplication and Division of Fractions.**

27. **C.** The correct solution is C. The line graph has the correct values for each roller coaster. **Skill: Interpreting Graphics.**

28. **C.** The correct solution is 7,000 votes because 28% of 25,000 is 7,000 voters. **Skill: Interpreting Graphics.**

29. **C.** The correct solution is 10 because the difference between boys and girls is 10 participants. **Skill: Interpreting Graphics.**

30. **D.** The builder began with having 1,350 screws between all three boxes. He used 150 from the first box, 75 from the second, and 270 from the third to use a total of 495 screws. This leaves him with 855 screws. **Skill: Multiplication and Division of Fractions.**

31. **A.** There are 80 cookies remaining because 120 ÷ 3 = 40, so her eldest grandchild ate 40 cookies. 120 − 40 = 80 cookies. **Skill: Multiplication and Division of Fractions.**

32. **B.** The correct solution is 18 because the equation simplifies to $2x = 36$ and $x = 18$. **Skill: Equations with One Variable.**

33. **A.** The correct solution is $3x^3 - 6x^2 + 8x + 1$.

$$(-2x^2 + 8x) + (3x^3 - 4x^2 + 1) = 3x^3 + (-2x^2 - 4x^2) + 8x + 1 = 3x^3 - 6x^2 + 8x + 1$$

Skill: Polynomials.

34. **B.** The correct answer is $1\frac{3}{8}$ because $\frac{11}{6} \div \frac{4}{3} = \frac{11}{6} \times \frac{3}{4} = \frac{33}{24} = 1\frac{9}{24} = 1\frac{3}{8}$. **Skill: Multiplication and Division of Fractions.**

35. **B.** The pharmacist will fill the prescription with 100 pills because 10 grams is equal to 10,000 milligrams. Since the pills are 100 milligrams of medicine, 10,000 mg of medicine ÷ 100 mg per pill = 100 pills. **Skill: Solving Real World Mathematical Problems.**

36. D. Use the following equation to convert Celsuis to Fahrenheit:

$$F = (\tfrac{9}{5})C + 32$$

Where $F = (\tfrac{9}{5}) \times 105°C + 32 = 221$. **Skill: Temperature and the Metric System.**

Section III. Science

1. B. The skin and linings of the internal organs are examples of epithelial tissue. **Skill: Organization of the Human Body.**

2. D. Neural tissue coordinates and controls many body activities. It is found in the brain and spinal cord. **Skill: Organization of the Human Body.**

3. D. Blood is responsible for transporting waste products to the liver, where they are excreted as bile from the liver or as urine by the kidneys. **Skill: Cardiovascular System.**

4. C. Deoxygenated blood returns from systemic circulation through the veins, superior vena cava (upper half of body) and inferior vena cava (lower half of body) and pours into the right atrium. **Skill: Cardiovascular System.**

5. C. The blood levels of certain chemicals, such as insulin, directly control the secretion of some hormones. **Skill: Endocrine System.**

6. A. Autocrine chemical signals include prostaglandin-like chemicals that are secreted in response to inflammation, which can indicate an infection. **Skill: Endocrine System.**

7. A. Monitoring blood glucose levels is a vital function of the endocrine system. **Skill: Endocrine System.**

8. D. The primary function of the oral cavity is to break up the food through mastication. **Skill: Gastrointestinal System.**

9. C. The sublingual salivary glands are found under the tongue. **Skill: Gastrointestinal System.**

10. B. A major function of the large intestine is to squeeze all excess water from waste material for the body to reuse it. **Skill: Gastrointestinal System.**

11. A. Between the nail bed and cuticle is the lunula. This is an area of white space that is lighter than the nail plate. **Skill: Integumentary System.**

12. B. The epidermis consists of either four or five layers. This depends on the part of the body where the epidermis is located. The soles of the feet and palms of the hand have five layers, and all other parts of the body, including the face, have four layers. **Skill: Integumentary System.**

13. B. When the skin is saggy and thin due to aging, fat stores in the hypodermis are depleted or have been redistributed to other places in the body. Targeting this area for correction may help reverse the sagging skin. **Skill: Integumentary System.**

14. A. The heart is composed of three layers, the middle of which is the myocardium. The myocardium contains cardiac muscle tissue. **Skill: Cardiovascular System.**

15. C. In this case, the pathogen slipped past patrolling macrophages, the second line of defense. **Skill: The Lymphatic System.**

16. A. All muscles are elastic because they are flexible. That is, they can recoil and shorten after being stretched. **Skill: Muscular System.**

17. C. Muscle fibers are synonymous with the term *muscle cells* because these fibers are specialized cells designed to help the skeletal muscle contract. **Skill: Muscular System.**

18. A. When a flexor muscle contracts, it causes a joint to bend. During this contraction, the extension muscle straightens, or elongates. **Skill: Muscular System.**

19. B. The occipital lobe is part of the cerebrum. It interprets visual stimuli and information that comes from the eyes. **Skill: The Nervous System.**

20. C. The hypothalamus is a structure found in the forebrain and is part of the limbic system. It helps regulate processes in the body using neural and chemical signaling. Chemical signaling via hormones is completed when the limbic system works with the endocrine system, specifically the pituitary gland. **Skill: The Nervous System.**

21. B. Schwann cells are a type of glial cells cell found in the PNS. They produce myelin sheaths that insulate the axon of a neuron. **Skill: The Nervous System.**

22. B. The myelin sheath is an insulating outer layer that surrounds the axon. This blanket-like structure not only protects the axon, but also increases transmission of electric signals. **Skill: The Nervous System.**

23. A. Newborn humans require a great deal of parental care. Visual tracking of objects usually begins around three months of age; puberty does not start for several years; and reproductive capability does not start until the end of puberty. **Skill: Reproductive System.**

24. B. After fertilization takes place, hormonal changes signal pregnancy. The key signaling hormones are released by the developing zygote. Puberty must be complete before fertilization can occur, and menstruation stops during pregnancy, but not due to menopause. **Skill: Reproductive System.**

25. D. The nose is part of the upper respiratory tract. Because it is the site where air enters the body, nose hairs help prevent airborne particles from entering the lungs. **Skill: The Respiratory System.**

26. A. Pulmonary ventilation is the first step in external respiration, during which air moves into and out of the lungs. **Skill: The Respiratory System.**

27. C. As the diaphragm changes shape and moves down, the rib cage moves out, creating suction that draws in air. This is the process of inspiration. **Skill: The Respiratory System.**

28. D. Bones of the lower extremities include the metatarsals, or foot bones. Metacarpals are hand bones. **Skill: Skeletal System.**

29. A. The pectoral girdle is made up of the scapula and the clavicle. There are 2 clavicles and 2 scapulas, which make up the 4 bones in the pectoral girdle. **Skill: Skeletal System.**

30. A. The short bones, such as the carpal and tarsal bones of the wrist and feet, provide support. They have less flexibility than other bone types. **Skill: Skeletal System.**

31. A. The bladder is a sac-like organ that stores urine after it travels through the ureter. Once the bladder reaches half full, the urine is emptied into the urethra and out of the body. **Skill: The Urinary System.**

32. A. The first process that occurs in the nephrons of the kidneys is glomerular filtration. This is where blood that flows from the renal arteries into the kidneys is initially filtered. Certain substances and water are reabsorbed into the bloodstream following filtration. **Skill: The Urinary System.**

33. B. The hydrogen atoms in a water molecule will hydrogen bond with oxygen atoms. This attraction contributes to both the charge of water and properties of water. **Skill: An Introduction to Biology.**

34. C. After pyruvate molecules from glycolysis are produced, these sugar molecules are used to make 2 ATP molecules, 6 carbon dioxide molecules, and 6 NADH molecules. While cellulose is a carbohydrate like glucose, it is not used to produce pyruvate. Electrons are created during oxidative phosphorylation. **Skill: An Introduction to Biology.**

35. A. Two ATP molecules are produced after glycolysis. **Skill: An Introduction to Biology.**

36. B. To be catabolic, the glycolytic pathway must involve the breakdown of glucose into smaller molecules (called pyruvate) and the release of energy (in the form of ATP). **Skill: An Introduction to Biology.**

37. C. Plant cells are autotrophs that harness energy from the sun and use it to make food. This process of using energy to make food is done with the help of photosynthesis. **Skill: Cell Structure, Function, and Type.**

38. D. The endoplasmic reticulum functions as the cell's transportation system. It helps shuttle proteins and other molecules around the cell. This structure is found in both animal and plant cells. **Skill: Cell Structure, Function, and Type.**

39. B. A difference between mitosis and meiosis is that meiosis requires two rounds of cell division. At the end of both rounds, four haploid daughter cells have been produced. **Skill: Cellular Reproduction, Cellular Respiration, and Photosynthesis.**

40. C. Fermentation is a metabolic process that produces ATP in the absence of oxygen. Thus, it is an anaerobic form of respiration. **Skill: Cellular Reproduction, Cellular Respiration, and Photosynthesis.**

41. D. Cell reproduction is the process where cells grow and differentiate to create offspring or new cells. When the skin is damaged, new skin cells are needed which are created through cell reproduction. **Skill: Cellular Reproduction, Cellular Respiration, and Photosynthesis**

42. B. After the DNA strand is separated, a complementary strand is assembled. **Skill: Genetics and DNA.**

43. A. Each offspring receives 1 allele for a particular trait from each parent. **Skill: Genetics and DNA.**

44. A. The RNA molecule is released into the cell for the next stage. **Skill: Genetics and DNA.**

45. C. The replication of DNA ends with a twisted strand called a double helix. **Skill: Genetics and DNA.**

46. D. Around the world, the metric system is the accepted system of units for recording and communicating values. **Skill: Designing an Experiment.**

47. B. After a hypothesis is formed, variables are created when experiments are designed to test the hypothesis. **Skill: Designing an Experiment.**

48. C. Looking at the products, 8 molecules of CO_2 have a total of 16 oxygen atoms, and 10 water molecules have a total of 10 oxygen atoms. Therefore, the products have a total of 26 oxygen atoms. This requires 13 molecules of O_2 in the reactants to get a total of 26 atoms of oxygen. $2C_4H_{10} + 13O_2 \rightarrow 8CO_2 + 10H_2O$ **Skill: Chemical Equations.**

49. B. Both atoms can be identified as neon because the atomic number, which equals the number of protons, is 10 for both. However, they have different masses. The mass of Atom Y can be determined by adding the numbers of protons and neutrons (10 + 12) to get 22, which is different from the mass of Atom X. Because they are the same element with different masses, Atom X and Atom Y are isotopes. **Skill: Scientific Notation.**

50. B. The number of protons determines the identity of the element. Regardless of the number of neutrons and electrons, any atom that has 15 protons is phosphorus. **Skill: Scientific Notation.**

51. A. As a result of this polar configuration, water molecules are attracted to themselves. This causes water to be cohesive. **Skill: Properties of Matter.**

52. C. As a result of osmosis, the concentration of free water molecules will equalize on both sides of the membrane. **Skill: Properties of Matter.**

53. C. Freezing is the change of a liquid to a solid. **Skill: Properties of Matter.**

Section IV. English and Language Usage

1. C. White House. The White House is capitalized because it is an important governmental building. **Skill: Capitalization.**

2. C. *He claimed, "My history presentation was great!"* Quotation marks enclose direct statements. **Skill: Punctuation.**

3. B. For most words ending in consonants, just add -s. **Skill: Spelling.**

4. C. *Family* and *area* are common nouns and should not be capitalized. **Skill: Nouns.**

5. B. The relative pronoun *who* introduces a clause that gives more information about the noun *Mrs. Sato*. **Skill: Pronouns.**

6. D. *First* is an adjective that describes the noun *house*. **Skill: Adjectives and Adverbs.**

7. B. *Yet* is a conjunction. **Skill: Conjunctions and Prepositions.**

8. B. *Offered* and *advised* are simple past tense verb forms. **Skill: Verbs and Verb Tenses.**

9. C. *The automobile* and *the personal computer* are both singular subjects connected by *or*, so they take a singular verb form. **Skill: Subject and Verb Agreement.**

10. B. The verb *wants* has the subject *she*. **Skill: Subject and Verb Agreement.**

11. B. In questions with pronouns *where* and *what*, the verb agrees with the noun or pronoun that follows it. *Everyone* is the subject of the first sentence. It is third person singular, so it takes the verb form *is*. *They* is the subject of the second sentence, and it takes the verb form *are*. **Skill: Subject and Verb Agreement.**

12. D. *And.* It is the only conjunction that fits within the context of the sentence. **Skill: Types of Clauses.**

13. A. *While her kids swam in the pool.* It is dependent because it does not express a complete thought and relies on the independent clause. The word *while* also signifies the beginning of a dependent clause. **Skill: Types of Clauses.**

14. D. The subordinate conjunction *because* combines the sentences and puts the focus on Tony preparing for his job interview. **Skill: Types of Sentences.**

15. D. This sentence combines the information using parallel structure. **Skill: Types of Sentences.**

16. B. This sentence correctly fixes the fragment. **Skill: Types of Sentences.**

17. C. *You'll be okay.* It is the most informal sentence because it has a contraction and informal vocabulary. **Skill: Formal and Informal Language.**

18. A. *Please send me a timely response.* It is the most polite and formal sentence of the four. **Skill: Formal and Informal Language.**

19. D. The word *hamper* has more than one meaning. **Skill: Context Clues and Multiple Meaning Words.**

20. C. The meaning of <u>buckle</u> in the context of this sentence is "to collapse or bend." **Skill: Context Clues and Multiple Meaning Words.**

21. A. The meaning of <u>cabinet</u> in this context is "a body of advisors to the president." The phrase "advised" helps you figure out which meaning of <u>cabinet</u> is being used. **Skill: Context Clues and Multiple Meaning Words.**

22. B. The meaning of <u>morose</u> in the context of this sentence is "glum." **Skill: Context Clues and Multiple Meaning Words.**

23. B. The meaning of <u>loquacious</u> in this context is "tending to talk a great deal." The phrase "droned on" helps you figure out the meaning of <u>loquacious</u>. **Skill: Context Clues and Multiple Meaning Words.**

24. A. The root *irasc* means "to be angry" and the suffix *-ible* means "able to be," so *irascible* means "easily angered." **Skill: Root Words, Prefixes, and Suffixes.**

25. C. The prefix *re-* means "again," and the root word *juven* means "young," so *rejuvenate* means "to make someone feel young again." **Skill: Root Words, Prefixes, and Suffixes.**

26. A. The root *klept* means "steal," so a *kleptomaniac* is someone who steals. **Skill: Root Words, Prefixes, and Suffixes.**

27. D. The suffix that means "one who loves" is *-phile* as in the word *bibliophile*. **Skill: Root Words, Prefixes, and Suffixes.**

28. C. The root that means "color" is *chrom* as in *monochromatic*. **Skill: Root Words, Prefixes, and Suffixes.**

TEAS Practice Exam 4

Section I. Reading

You have 64 minutes to complete 53 questions.

Read the paragraph and answer questions 1-5.

The theater was packed. The audience watched with rapt attention as the characters lost their homes, their jobs, their sense of security, even their most basic beliefs. A few characters managed to save a family member. Most kept small keepsakes in their pockets. But by the end, they had almost nothing left of the world before disaster struck. When the show was over, the audience filed out smiling. After all, there's nothing more fun than the end of the world—as long as it's fictional.

1. **Which sentence best describes the main idea of this paragraph?**

   A. There is a new disaster movie in the theaters.

   B. People who experience disasters must be very strong.

   C. For some reason, people find disaster movies entertaining.

   D. There is something wrong with people who like disaster movies.

2. **Which term best describes the role of the final sentence in this paragraph?**

   A. Implied idea

   B. Topic sentence

   C. Supporting detail

   D. Introductory sentence

3. **Which sentence states the most important effect of the author's decision to save the topic sentence for last?**

   A. It avoids offending.

   B. It distracts the reader.

   C. It changes the subject.

   D. It maximizes the impact.

4. **If the author wanted to expand this paragraph into a longer essay claiming that human beings are naturally violent, what supporting detail should appear in further paragraphs?**

   A. A review of the latest disaster movie

   B. An argument for censorship to end violence

   C. Eamples of bravery and generosity in disaster movies

   D. Examples of violent entertainment throughout history

5. **If the author wanted to expand this paragraph into a longer essay claiming that disaster movies serve a positive function, what supporting detail should appear in further paragraphs?**

   A. A review of the latest disaster movie

   B. An argument for censorship to end violence

   C. Examples of bravery and generosity in disaster movies

   D. Examples of violent entertainment throughout history

A high school student is presenting research on how gender affects participation in her political science class. Study the graphic elements below and answer questions 6-8.

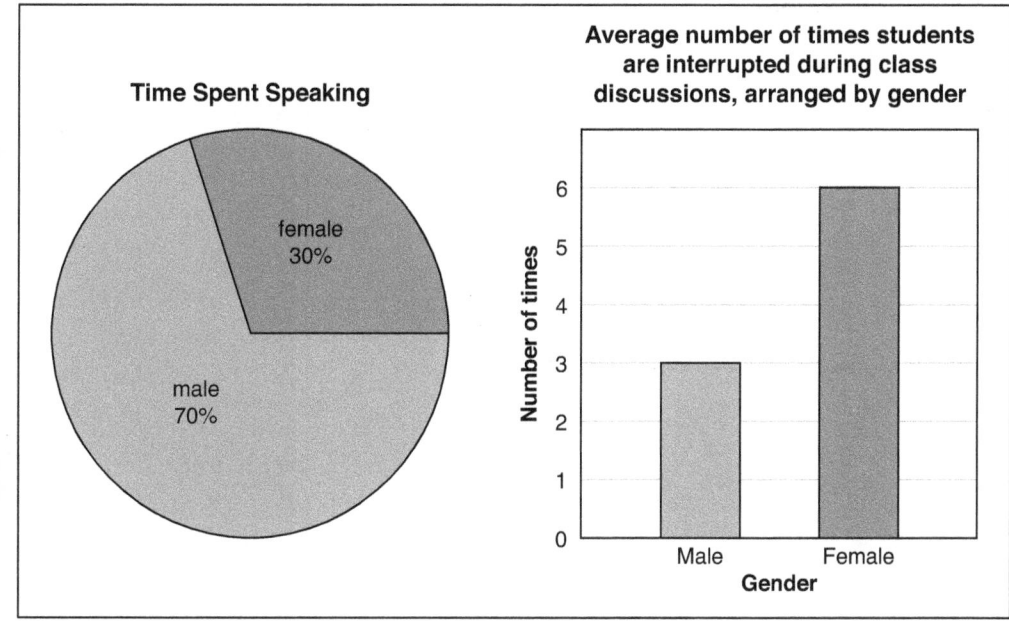

6. Male students spend _____ of class time speaking.

   A. 3%   C. 30%

   B. 6%   D. 70%

7. Which statement accurately describes the average number of interruptions during each class discussion?

   A. Male students are interrupted an average of six times.

   B. Female students are interrupted an average of six times.

   C. Male students interrupt others an average of three times.

   D. Female students interrupt others an average of three times.

8. Which argument does the information in the graphs best support?

   A. Female students do not have as many ideas about political science as male students.

   B. The class should make a greater effort to give students of both genders a fair chance to speak.

   C. Contrary to popular belief, male students face greater gender discrimination in school settings.

   D. There is no substantial difference between male and female students' class participation in discussions.

9. A(n) _____ main idea is suggested, not stated outright.

   A. explicit   C. persuasive

   B. implied   D. informational

Study the flowchart below and answer questions 10-11.

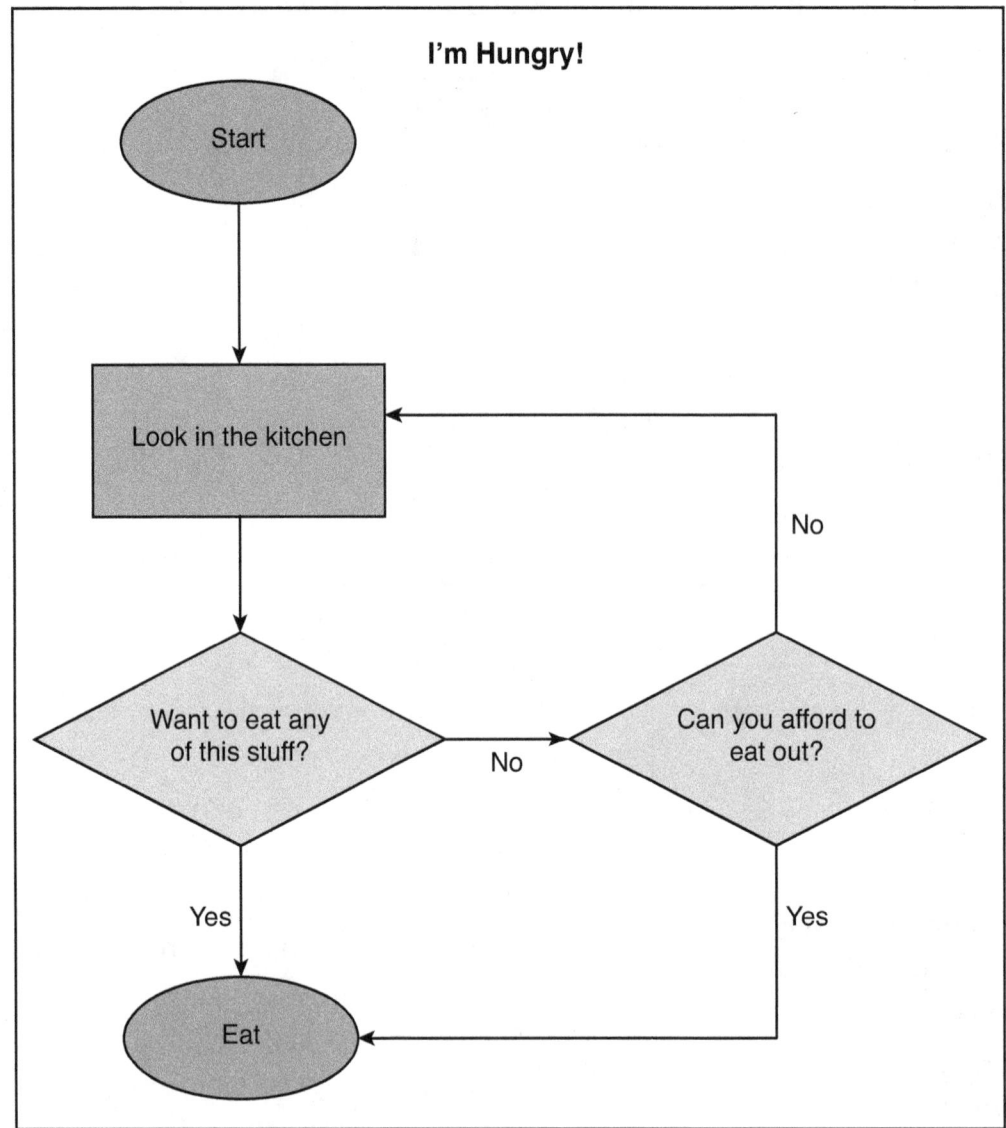

10. **What is the first thing the chart asks you to do if you are hungry?**

    A. Eat.

    B. Look in the kitchen.

    C. Consider whether you can afford to eat out.

    D. Consider whether you want to eat what you have.

11. **According to the flowchart, what do you need to do if you cannot afford to eat out?**

    A. Grow a garden.

    B. Get a better job.

    C. Buy a recipe book.

    D. Find food in the kitchen.

12. **What are graphic elements in a text?**

    A. Ideas arranged sequentially

    B. Main ideas restated differently

    C. Information presented visually

    D. White space between paragraphs

13. **Which of the following statements accurately describes a summary?**

    A. A summary makes a judgment about the original text.

    B. A summary leaves out the main idea of the original text.

    C. A summary restates implicit ideas from the original text.

    D. A summary copies words and phrases from the original text.

14. **What type of graphic element would best show which proportion of the economy is made up of manufacturing, agriculture, services, and so on?**

    A. Diagram   C. Bar graph

    B. Pie chart   D. Flowchart

15. **If an essay includes a quotation to back up a point, the writer does not need to:**

    A. identify the source of the quote.

    B. restate the quote in different words.

    C. include a properly formatted citation.

    D. explain how the quote supports the point.

16. **Which structure would most likely fit a paragraph describing the 2008 financial crisis and its consequences in the job market?**

    A. Sequential   C. Cause/effect

    B. Descriptive   D. Compare/
                           contrast

17. **When you're considering which of two words to use in an essay and you have no strong reason to do otherwise, you should choose the:**

    A. simplest one.

    B. prettiest one.

    C. most positive one.

    D. most complicated one.

18. **What is a transition in writing?**

    A. A well-defended opinion

    B. An organizational scheme

    C. A connecting word or phrase

    D. A piece of evidence with a citation

19. **Read the following sentences:**

    Winston Smith grows increasingly ambitious in his acts of rebellion against Big Brother and the Party. _____ he is convinced from the beginning that he will be caught.

    Which transition would *best* fit into the space above?

    A. Similarly   C. For example

    B. Previously   D. Nevertheless

20. **Read the sentences below.**

    Simon decided to play football all day instead of study for his math test. He received a poor grade.

    Which word or phrase, if inserted at the beginning of sentence two, would effectively transition between these two ideas?

    A. Likewise   C. As a result

    B. However   D. For example

Read the passage below and answer questions 21-26.

The train was the most amazing thing ever even though it didn't go "choo choo." The toddler pounded on the railing of the bridge and supplied the sound herself. "Choo choo! Choo choooooo!" she shouted as the train cars whizzed along below.

In the excitement, she dropped her favorite binky.

Later, when she noticed the binky missing, all the joy went out of the world. The wailing could be heard three houses down. The toddler's usual favorite activities were garbage—even waving to Hank the garbage man, which she refused to do, so that Hank went away looking mildly hurt. It was clear the little girl would never, ever, ever recover from her loss.

Afterward, she played at the park.

21. **Which adjectives best describe the tone of the passage?**
    A. Ironic, angry
    B. Earnest, angry
    C. Ironic, humorous
    D. Earnest, humorous

22. **Which sentence from the passage is clearly ironic?**
    A. "Choo choo! Choo choooooo!" she shouted as the train cars whizzed along below.
    B. Later, when she noticed the binky missing, all the joy went out of the world.
    C. The wailing could be heard three houses down.
    D. Afterward, she played at the park.

23. **The author of the passage first establishes the ironic tone by:**
    A. describing the child's trip to play at the park.
    B. calling the train "the most amazing thing ever."
    C. pretending that the child can make the sounds "choo choooo!"
    D. claiming inaccurately that the lost binky was the child's "favorite."

24. **Reread the following sentence:**

    It was clear the little girl would never, ever, ever recover from her loss.

    Which adjective could describe an effective reader's mood when reading this line in the context of the passage?
    A. Amused   C. Horrified
    B. Worried   D. Jubilant

25. **Which word or phrase does *not* function as a transition in the passage?**
    A. Later   C. Afterward
    B. Below   D. In the excitement

26. The transitions "later" and "afterward" link ideas in the passage by showing:

    A. when events happen in time.

    B. how certain ideas contrast.

    C. examples that illustrate ideas.

    D. cause-and-effect relationships.

27. The author's _____ is his or her general outlook or set of opinions about the subject.

    A. purpose

    C. main idea

    B. reasoning

    D. point of view

28. What is the most likely purpose of a cookbook full of Mediterranean recipes?

    A. To decide

    C. To persuade

    B. To inform

    D. To entertain

Read the passage and answer questions 29-33.

Our survey revealed a broad pattern of unconscious bias against minority students on majority-white college campuses. First, a startlingly high proportion of minority respondents, 83%, reported that they often or sometimes felt marginalized or overlooked by members of their broader campus communities.

In a follow-up telephone interview, Aida Green, an African American sophomore at Standmore University in Iowa, said that students in campus common areas often asked her questions like, "Where are you visiting from?" Although these encounters typically take a friendly tone, Green said the underlying message is clear: her community fails to recognize her as a member. When asked why this matters, Green sounded frustrated. "I see people's eyes pass over me when they're forming study groups. White kids get asked; I have to put myself forward." She sighed. "And that's if I know an opportunity exists. I'm always wondering what I could be doing to get ahead that I'm not doing because nobody thought to tell me I can."

Similar patterns existed in other minority students' survey comments and interviews. The most common type of statement was a sentiment of fatigue; students feel exhausted by the effort to insert themselves into groups that unconsciously exclude them. And many students echoed Green's worry that they may be missing out on opportunities. Clarity Ferrer, a black Puerto Rican senior at Northeastern College of Vermont, was certain she had been overlooked: "My own sorority sisters started holding informal lunches with alumni to talk about jobs and internships, and they didn't invite me the whole first quarter. All the other seniors got told about it. But me? They forgot."

29. What is the primary purpose of the passage?

    A. To annoy

    C. To persuade

    B. To inform

    D. To entertain

30. **With which statement would the authors of the passage most likely agree?**

    A. Clarity Ferrer's sorority sisters probably excluded her on purpose for a reason that had nothing to do with race.

    B. Unconscious racism on college campuses may be a cause of income gaps between white and minority college graduates.

    C. Even if minority students encounter unconscious bias, they do not suffer much because affirmative action helps them.

    D. White students at majority-white campuses nationwide are actively coordinating an attempt to keep minority students down.

31. **Which sentence expresses an argument supported by the evidence in the passage?**

    A. Campus communities should require students to undergo training to address their unconscious biases.

    B. Colleges should offer minority students more opportunities to rest because racism makes them tired.

    C. Minority students should be offered training and support so they get better at enduring slight hints of racism.

    D. If we can end the unconscious marginalization of minority college students, racism in the United States will be solved.

32. **The authors most likely included Aida Green's comments in order to:**

    A. show that marginalization is one of a constellation of problems, most of which are not clear from survey data.

    B. add an emotional component to the statistical information that 83% of minority students feel marginalized.

    C. appeal to the reader's reason by adding statistical data to back up an opinion shared by many survey respondents.

    D. distract readers from the main idea in order to trick them into believing an argument that is not sufficiently supported.

33. **The authors most likely include the statistic about the percentage of minority students who feel marginalized in order to:**

    A. show that experiences with marginalization are widespread.

    B. scare readers into thinking they may be unconscious racists.

    C. provide a counterpoint to an argument in favor of bias training.

    D. distract from the fact that 17% of minority students did not feel marginalized.

Read the following passage and answer questions 34-36.

Every time I visit the bookstore, I find a new science fiction title about post-apocalyptic survivors taking refuge in New York City's subway tunnels. Some of these survival stories are fun to read, but they have a pesky plausibility problem: if society collapses, those subway tunnels won't be there anymore—at least not for long. On a typical day in a functioning New York City, a crew of engineers works around the clock to pump about 13 million gallons of water out of the subway system, and a major rain event pushes that number up fast. What happens if you take the engineers—and the electricity to work the sump pumps—out of the equation? The first big storm will flood those tunnels, probably for good. At that point, any survivors left underground will have to grow gills or head for the surface.

34. **Which of the following is the best title for this passage?**

   A. A Visit to a Bookstore

   B. The Science of Growing Gills

   C. A Refuge in Fiction, but Not in Fact

   D. The Best Science Fiction of the Year

35. **Which graphic element would most clearly illustrate the author's point?**

   A. A schematic showing the depth and volume of all of New York City's subway tunnels

   B. A graph comparing the ridership of New York City's subways with those of other major American cities

   C. A table showing how much water runs through the New York City subway system in varying conditions

   D. A New York City subway map showing emergency exits and detailing procedures for exiting the system during a flood

36. **Which information would belong in a sidebar alongside this text?**

   A. An illustration showing how a family of people might look if they all had gills behind their ears

   B. A description of a subway's electrified third rail and an explanation of how it works to power the train

   C. A list of science fiction novels about people living in subway tunnels in a post-apocalyptic world

   D. A description of the job qualifications of a subway engineer who works the pumps to keep the tunnels functional

37. **Which of the following is *not* a function of text features?**

   A. Introducing the topic

   B. Emphasizing a concept

   C. Making the theme explicit

   D. Providing peripheral information

38. If a map does not have a compass, north is:

   A. up.   C. right.
   B. down.   D. left.

39. What is a bias?

   A. A preconceived and sometimes unfair belief
   B. A person or group that often faces prejudice
   C. An unstated idea that underlies an argument
   D. A sweeping statement that may not always be true

40. A particularly harmful kind of bias is called a(n):

   A. opinion.   C. assumption.
   B. stereotype.   D. over-generalization.

41. Which of the following is *not* clearly a form of faulty reasoning?

   A. Either/or fallacy
   B. Circular reasoning
   C. An overgeneralization
   D. A statement of opinion

42. Which sentence does *not* display gender bias?

   A. Since the dawn of humankind, man has wondered about the stars.
   B. Since the dawn of mankind, people have wondered about the stars.
   C. Since the dawn of humankind, people have wondered about the stars.
   D. Since the dawn of humankind, the stars have captured man's imagination.

43. Read the following sentence.

   A nurse should not divulge personal information about her patients.

   Which revision eliminates gender bias?

   A. A nurse should not divulge personal information about his patients.
   B. Nurses should not divulge personal information about their patients.
   C. A patient should not have his persona information revealed by a medical professional.
   D. A nurse should not divulge personal information about her patients regardless of gender.

44. Which sentence does *not* display gender bias?

   A. The parent who feeds her infant organic foods cares for her infant's physical growth.
   B. The parent who feeds his infant organic foods cares for his infant's physical growth.
   C. The parent who feeds an infant organic foods cares for the infant's physical growth.
   D. The parent who feeds their infant organic foods cares for her infant's physical growth.

45. Which source would provide the *least* credible information to a researcher interested in studying changes in parenting techniques over the past forty years?

   A. An op-ed piece in today's newspaper on the hardships of being a parent of an adolescent

   B. A currently published interview with a pediatrician on the benefits of positive discipline

   C. A book published in 1985 about best practices in raising your child

   D. A recent article in *Parenting Magazine* about parenting in the 1980s vs. today

46. An art major finds a video presentation of a group of people commenting on the works of a famous artist she has been studying. She is deciding if it is a credible source. Which detail about the video, if true, would *not* give her reason to trust the video?

   A. The video was filmed within the past two years.

   B. One of the speakers is a renowned Ivy League Art History professor.

   C. Real paintings of the artists' work are shown.

   D. The video is highly edited, and some speakers are cut off mid-sentence.

Read the following passage and answer questions 47-49.

Are you tired of your children not listening to you? Do they seem distracted every time you ask them to do something? Are you met with a glossy-eyed stare every time you say something to them? Part of the problem is too much screen time.

Technology has its benefits, but it does a lot to ruin our children's focus. There are too many flashes of light, too many colors, too many hyperlinks to navigate – it's a wonder our children can even focus at all!

Limiting your children's screen time would do wonders for them. Make more time to have face-to-face conversations. This will allow your children to actually practice good listening and communication skills. Hand them a book! This will help them sit still and focus on one thing for a period of time.

Technology won't be going away anytime soon, but you can set limits for your children to help them focus, listen, and better engage with you.

47. This article is written for:

   A. parents.   C. teachers.

   B. children.   D. policymakers.

48. The author of this article assumes that:

   A. parents are frustrated by their children not listening to them.

   B. parents are on screens more than their children are.

   C. children do not like to be told what to do by their parents.

   D. children would rather talk and read books than be on screens.

49. Which conclusion is *not* supported by the article?

    A. The author thinks kids are on their screens too much.

    B. The author thinks technology is negatively impacting children.

    C. The author thinks parents do not know how to discipline their children.

    D. The author thinks parents need to do more to help draw kids away from technology.

50. A student finds an online video of a conference presentation related to her scientific research topic and wants to decide if it is credible. Which detail about the video, if true, would *not* give her more reason to trust the video?

    A. The conference took place in the last year.

    B. The speaker makes highly emotional arguments.

    C. The conference host is clearly identified and reputable.

    D. The speaker is a Harvard professor in a field related to the research.

51. Which term describes the most likely structure of an essay about the similarities and differences between World War I and World War II?

    A. Technical   C. Cause/effect

    B. Expository   D. Compare/contrast

52. Which of the following is an example of persuasive writing?

    A. A user manual

    B. A history book

    C. An op-ed article

    D. An autobiography

53. What are the two basic genres that encompass all of literature?

    A. Fable and myth

    B. Fiction and nonfiction

    C. Technical and expository

    D. Sequence and description

SECTION II. MATHEMATICS

You will have 54 minutes to complete 36 questions.

. The double line chart shows the number of points scored and points given up by a
basketball team over the first 10 games. Which statement is true?

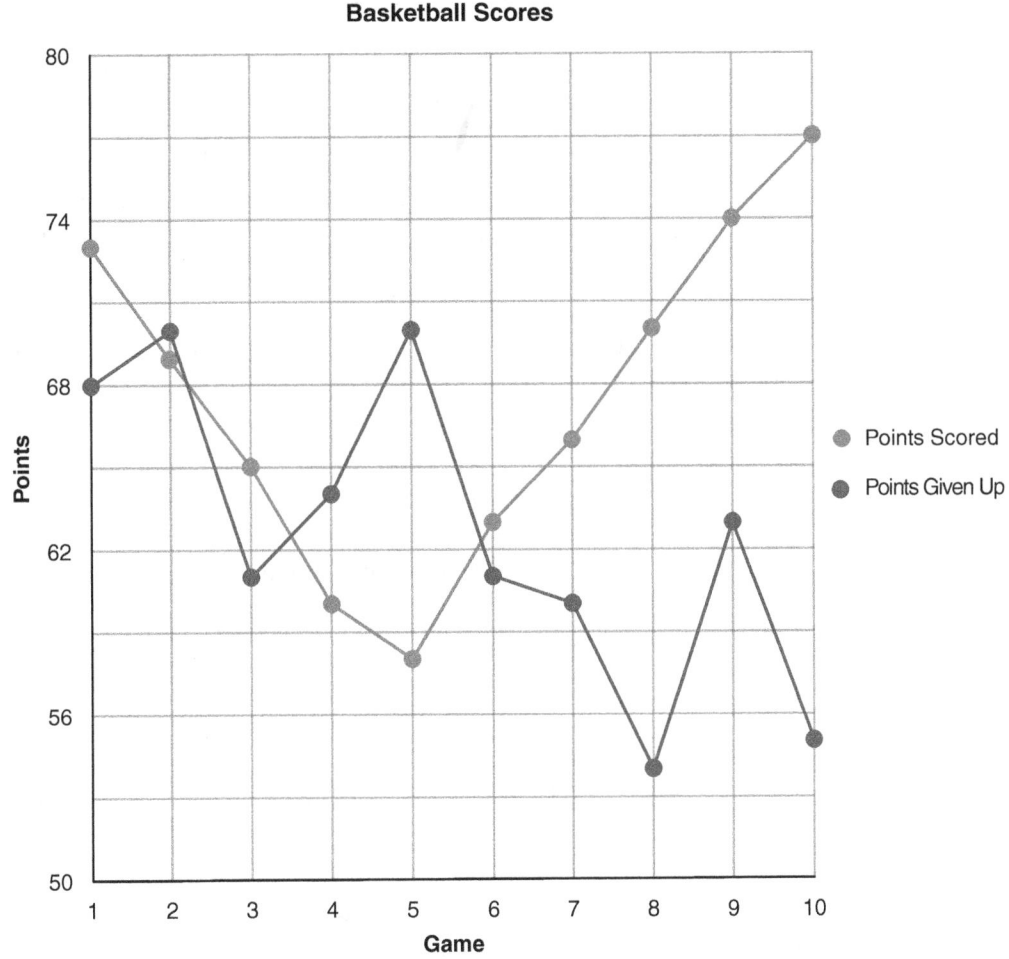

A. The team scored more than 62 points in
a majority of games and gave up fewer
than 62 points in a majority of games.

B. The team scored more than 65 points in
a majority of games and gave up fewer
than 65 points in a majority of games.

C. The team scored more than 68 points in
a majority of games and gave up fewer
than 68 points in a majority of games.

D. The team scored more than 70 points in
a majority of games and gave up fewer
than 65 points in a majority of games.

2. $\frac{15}{10} - \frac{2}{3}$

   A. $\frac{1}{2}$ C. $\frac{5}{6}$

   B. $\frac{13}{7}$ D. $1\frac{3}{10}$

3. If 35% of a cattle herd is Ayrshire and the rest is Jersey, and it has 195 Jerseys, how many cattle are in the herd?

   A. 230   C. 300

   B. 263   D. 557

4. What is the product of 3:2 and 5:6?

   A. 4:5   C. 5:4

   B. 1:1   D. 9:5

5. How many men does a company employ if it has 420 employees and 35% are women?

   A. 35   C. 273

   B. 147   D. 420

6. Find the median from the dot plot.

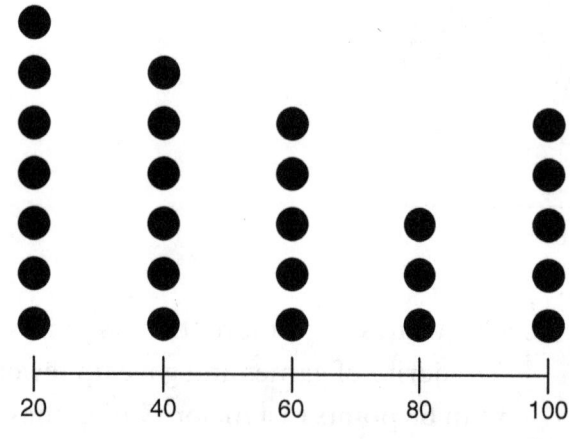

   A. 40   C. 60

   B. 50   D. 70

7. Henry leaves work driving at an average speed of 50 miles per hour. If he needs to travel 30 miles to his home, how long will it take him to arrive?

   A. 36 minutes   C. 34 minutes

   B. 25 minutes   D. 40 minutes

8. Convert 2 feet to centimeters. (Note: 1 inch is equal to 2.54 centimeters.)

   A. 30.49 centimeters   C. 50.49 centimeters

   B. 40.98 centimeters   D. 60.98 centimeters

9. Which expression is different from the others?

   A. 4:9   C. 44%

   B. 0.44   D. $\frac{9}{4}$

10. Perform the operation.

   $(8x + 2xy - 4y) + (-7x - 3xy + 2y)$

   A. $x + xy - 2y$ C. $x - xy + 2y$

   B. $x - xy - 2y$ D. $x + xy + 2y$

11. Write 145.5% as a decimal.

   A. 1.455   C. 145.5

   B. 14.55   D. 1455

12. Convert 75°F to the Celsius scale. (Note: °C = 5 _ 9(°F − 32).)

   A. 60°C   C. 41°C

   B. 77°C   D. 24°C

13. Alan makes a $518 car payment every month for 6 years. If he never made a down payment, how much money did he pay for the car in total?

   A. $36,260   C. $36,960

   B. $35,224   D. $37,296

14. The table shows the temperature in Fahrenheit degrees for two cities the first ten days of December. Select the correct line graph for this data.

Day	1	2	3	4	5	6	7	8	9	10
City 1	25	18	34	29	32	26	19	15	12	7
City 2	14	20	22	18	20	18	14	9	8	11

A.
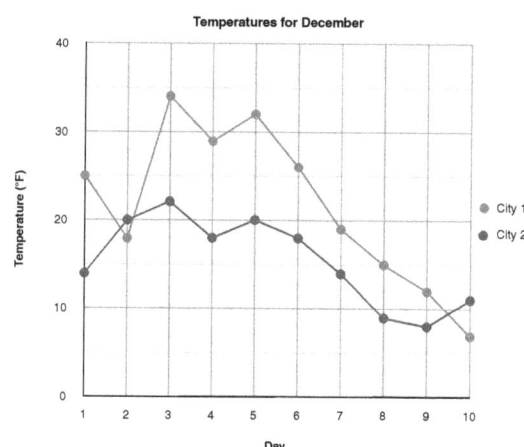

C.
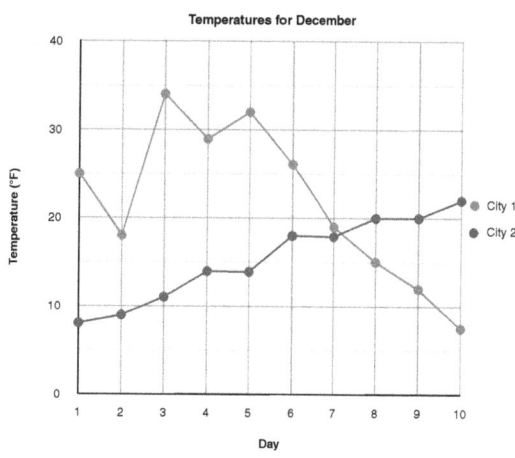

B.
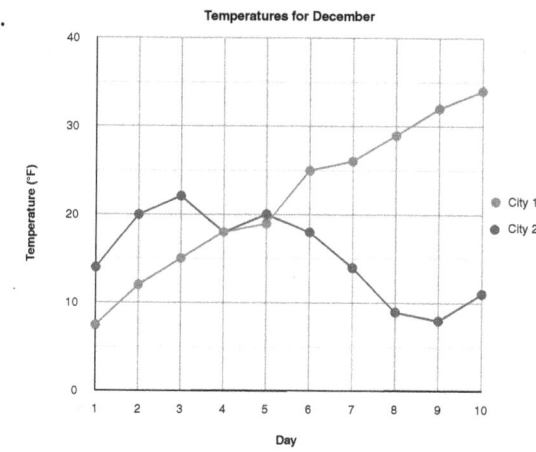

D.
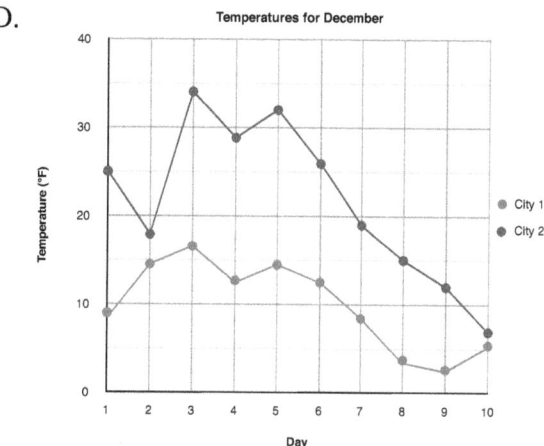

15. Write $83.\overline{3}\%$ as a decimal.

   A. $8.\overline{3}$

   B. $0.8\overline{3}$

   C. $0.08\overline{3}$

   D. 0.0083

16. Convert 0.5 kiloliter to milliliters. (Note: 1 kiloliter is equal to 1,000,000 milliliters.)

   A. 50,000 milliliters

   B. 500,000 milliliters

   C. 5,000,000 milliliters

   D. 50,000,000 milliliters

17. Hannah works at a company that pays her a salary of $2,150 every three weeks. If she works for an entire year, minus one work week because she took time off without paid leave, what is her estimated salary?

   A. $37,370

   B. $38,700

   C. $36,550

   D. $34,400

18. The bar chart shows the number of items collected for a charity drive. Which statement is true for the bar chart?

Items Collected

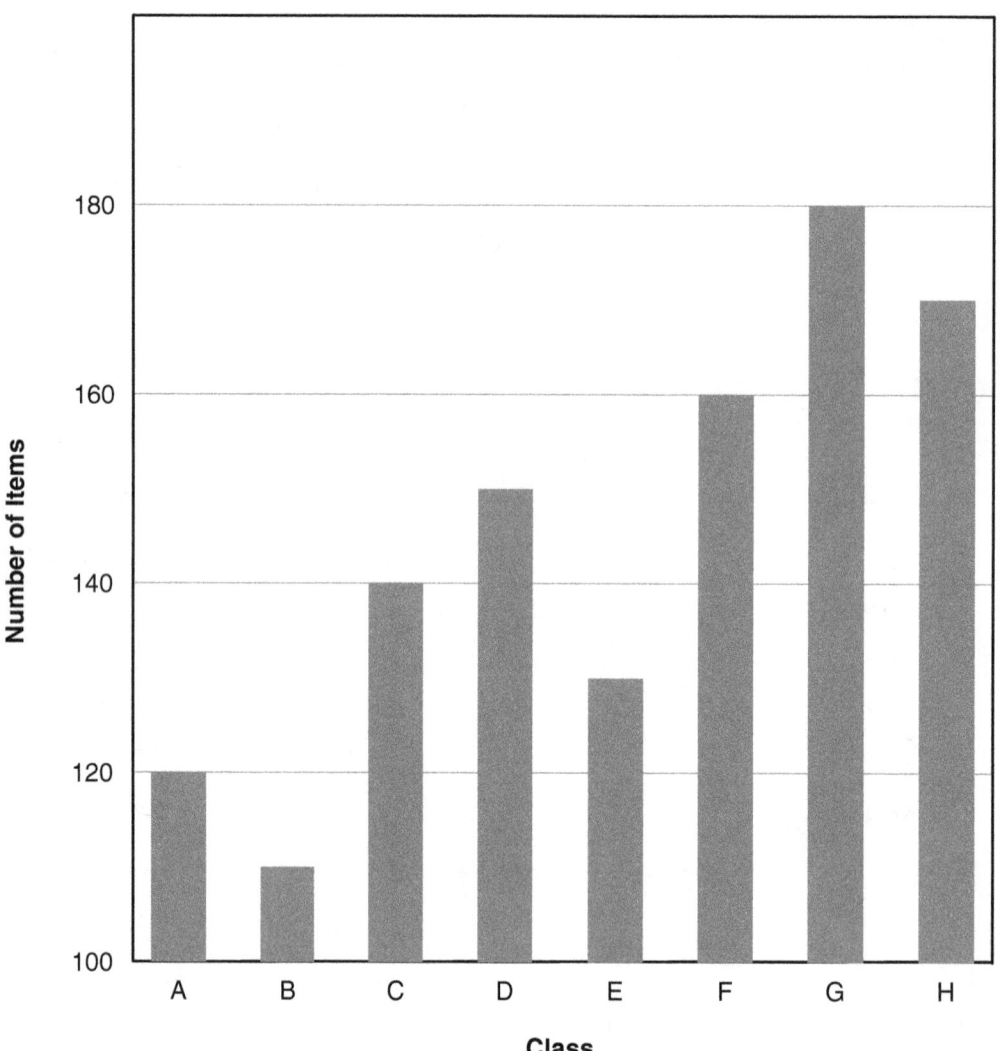

A. Classes F, G, and H each collected more than 150 items.

B. Classes D, F, and G each collected more than 150 items.

C. Classes C, D, and E each collected more than 140 items.

D. Classes A, B, and C each collected more than 140 items.

19. Solve for the value of *y* when *x* = 9.

$$y = (x^2 + 3) \div 3$$

A. 21 C. 9

B. 7 D. 28

20. $5\frac{1}{2} \times \frac{7}{8}$

A. $4\frac{3}{10}$ C. $5\frac{7}{16}$

B. $4\frac{13}{16}$ D. $5\frac{7}{10}$

21. $1\frac{1}{2} \times 2\frac{1}{3}$

    A. $3\frac{1}{6}$ C. $3\frac{1}{4}$

    B. $3\frac{1}{5}$ D. $3\frac{1}{2}$

22. Solve the equation for the unknown.

    $\frac{3}{4}(x + 3) - 2 = 3 - \frac{2}{3}(x + 1)$

    A. $\frac{6}{5}$ C. $\frac{8}{5}$

    B. $\frac{25}{17}$ D. $\frac{28}{17}$

23. Write $\frac{7}{9}$ as a percent.

    A. $0.\overline{7}\%$ C. $77.\overline{7}\%$

    B. $7.\overline{7}\%$ D. $777.\overline{7}\%$

24. Solve for x.

    $(4 - 2)x = 64 \div 4$

    A. 8   C. 4

    B. 2   D. 16

25. The combined area of two identical rectangular tarps is 448 square feet. What is the length in feet of one tarp if the width is 14 feet? (Note: A = length × width.)

    A. 8   C. 24

    B. 16   D. 32

26. In a backyard, $\frac{1}{6}$ of the yard is a garden, $\frac{2}{5}$ is landscaped, and $\frac{1}{3}$ is for play. How much of the yard is available for other use?

    A. $\frac{1}{10}$ C. $\frac{13}{15}$

    B. $\frac{2}{15}$ D. $\frac{9}{10}$

27. A woman rents a 1-bedroom apartment from her landlord at $850 a month. She finds out her friend has a 2-bedroom apartment in the same building for $1,000 a month. How much more money a year does it cost her friend to have the second bedroom?

    A. $1,500   C. $1,200

    B. $1,600   D. $1,800

28. A shoebox in the shape of a right rectangular prism has a surface area of 400 square inches. What is the length in inches if the other two dimensions are 8 inches and 14 inches? (Note: $SA = 2lw + 2lh + 2hw$.)

    A. 2   C. 4

    B. 3   D. 5

29. Solve the equation for the unknown.

    $\frac{x}{4} + 8 = 6$

    A. −8   C. 2

    B. −2   D. 8

30. Convert 16 gallons to liters. (Note: 1 gallon is equal to 3.79 liters.)

    A. 12.21 liters   C. 58.28 liters

    B. 19.79 liters   D. 60.64 liters

31. A circle has a circumference of 72 centimeters. Find the radius to the nearest tenth of a centimeter. Use 3.14 for π.

    A. 6.3   C. 17.2

    B. 11.5   D. 22.9

32. A mixture for a cake has various parts. Select the correct circle graph for the data.

Part	Eggs	Water	Oil	Mixture	Vanilla
Parts	2	3	2	7	1

A.

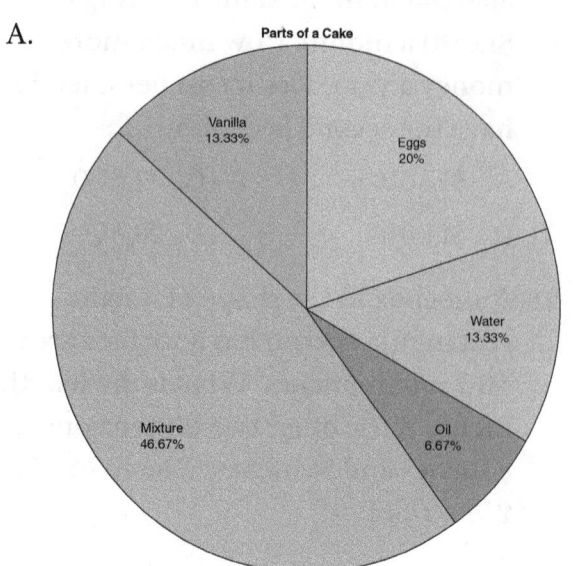

C.

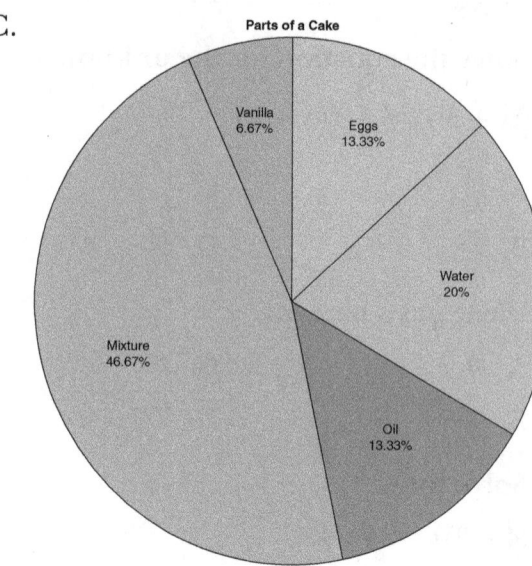

B.

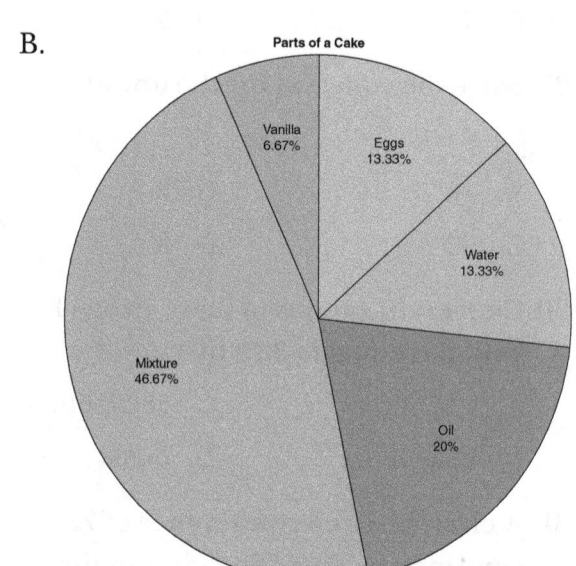

D.

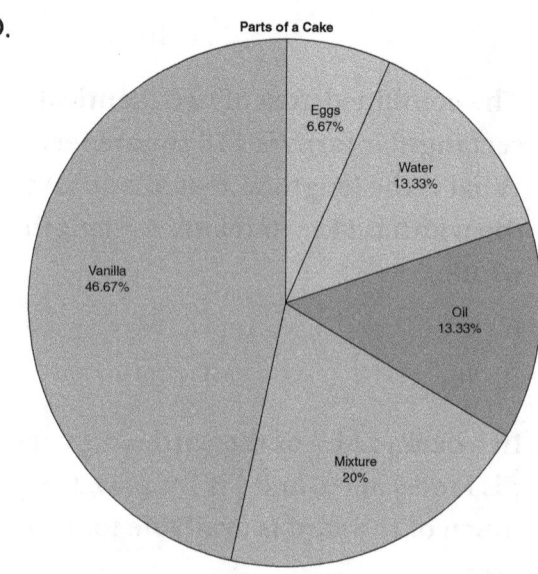

33. The data below shows a class's quiz scores out of 20 points.

5, 5, 6, 7, 8, 8, 9, 10, 11, 12, 13, 14, 15, 15, 16, 18, 18, 19, 20, 20

Select a box plot for the data.

A.

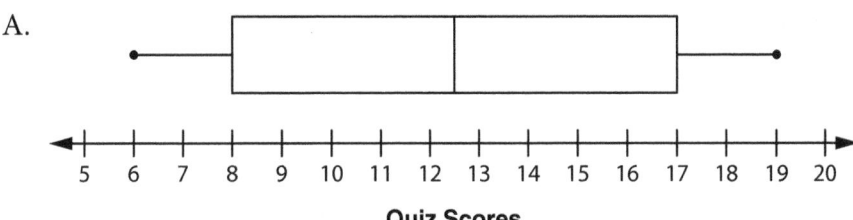

Quiz Scores

B.

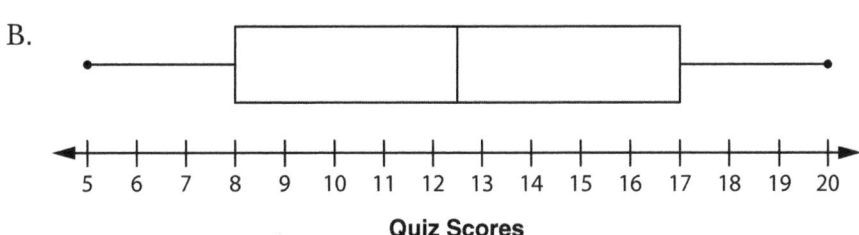

Quiz Scores

C.

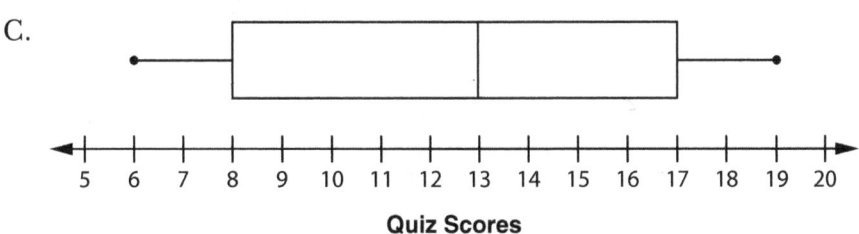

Quiz Scores

D.

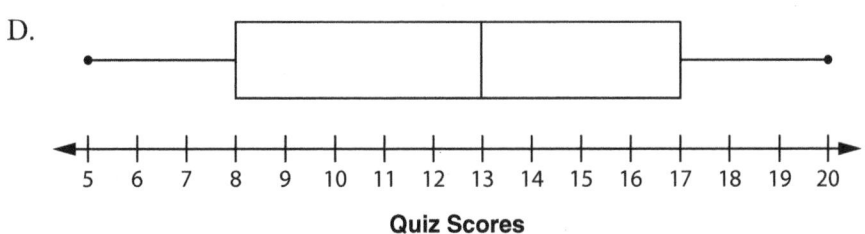

Quiz Scores

34. A cube has a side length of 15 millimeters. What is the volume in cubic millimeters? (Note: The volume of a cube is $V = $ length × width × height.)

   A. 45   C. 3,375

   B. 1,350   D. 6,750

35. Solve the equation for the unknown, y.

   $Ax + By = C$

   A. $y = C + Ax$ C. $y = \frac{C + Ax}{B}$

   B. $y = C - Ax$ D. $y = \frac{C - Ax}{B}$

36. A nurse needs to administer 0.5 grams of medicine to a patient every hour until the patient has received 2500 milligrams (mg) worth of medicine. If the nurse is prompt on her care, how many times will nurse give the patient medicine? (Note: 1 gram is equal to 1,000 mg.)

   A. 1   C. 7

   B. 10   D. 5

SECTION III. SCIENCE

You have 63 minutes to complete 53 questions.

1. Which of the following levels of body organization involves the interactions between atoms and molecules?
   A. Cell
   B. Chemical
   C. Organ
   D. Tissue

2. What anatomical term means "away from the surface"?
   A. Anterior
   B. Deep
   C. Proximal
   D. Ventral

3. Which term is synonymous with *posterior*?
   A. Dorsal
   B. Inferior
   C. Proximal
   D. Superior

4. What happens after blood coagulation?
   A. Platelet plug forms.
   B. Fibrin mesh is created.
   C. Blood vessels contract.
   D. Wounded site is closed.

5. What is the densest component of blood?
   A. Plasma
   B. Platelets
   C. Leukocytes
   D. Reddish mass

6. An area on a person's arm becomes inflamed. What type of response does this indicate?
   A. Autocrine
   B. Neuromodulator
   C. Paracrine
   D. Pheromone

7. What are the building blocks of carbohydrates?
   A. Glycerols
   B. Fatty acids
   C. Amino acids
   D. Monosaccharides

8. What is the first enzyme that functions in the digestive system?
   A. Amylase
   B. Lactase
   C. Maltase
   D. Sucrase

9. What organ of the digestive system stores concentrated bile?
   A. Gallbladder
   B. Liver
   C. Pancreas
   D. Stomach

10. Which is the point where the small and large intestines meet?
    A. anus
    B. appendix
    C. cecum
    D. colon

11. What is the outer layer of the nail called?
    A. Bed
    B. Matrix
    C. Plate
    D. Shaft

12. What segment of the electrocardiogram is associated with atrial systole?
    A. P wave
    B. S wave
    C. ST segment
    D. QRS complex

13. How many types of neuroglia are found in the CNS?
    A. 2
    B. 4
    C. 11
    D. 17

14. **Which of the following is part of the axial skeleton?**

    A. Carpals   C. Patella

    B. Femur   D. Skull

15. **As a person ages, the body produces fewer _____.**

    A. B cells   C. helper T cells

    B. B and T cells   D. macrophage cells

16. **Which organ of the urinary system filters blood?**

    A. Bladder   C. Ureter

    B. Kidney   D. Urethra

17. **What is the A-band?**

    A. Middle region of a sarcomere

    B. Attachment site for actin filaments

    C. Area consisting of thick and thin filaments

    D. Dark band location in the middle of I-bands

18. **Which structure is found between skull bones?**

    A. Tendon   C. Fibrous joint

    B. Ligament   D. Cartilaginous joint

19. **The muscular system is best known for:**

    A. promoting bone stabilization.

    B. generating heat energy for the body.

    C. controlling when muscle fibers contract.

    D. decreasing rhythmic movement of the heart.

20. **Which of the following are transmitted during a neural impulse?**

    A. Sodium ions

    B. Calcium ions

    C. Electric signals

    D. Chemical signals

21. **After calcium ions flow into the presynaptic membrane of a neuron,**

    A. vesicles undergo exocytosis.

    B. an action potential is established.

    C. potassium ions enter the axon bulb.

    D. neurotransmitters bind to receptors.

22. **What is the synaptic cleft?**

    A. Space between two neurons

    B. Site where calcium channels open

    C. Region filled with cerebrospinal fluid

    D. Location where neurons bind to muscle cells

23. **What happens if fertilization does not occur?**

    A. the unfertilized ovum returns to the ovary

    B. the unfertilized ovum remains in the Fallopian tube

    C. the unfertilized ovum passes out of the body during menstruation

    D. the unfertilized ovum implants into the endometrial lining of the uterus

24. **Which of the following correctly orders the route of nourishment from mother to fetus?**

    A. Placenta umbilical uterus

    B. Umbilical uterus placenta

    C. Uterus placenta umbilical

    D. Placenta uterus umbilical

25. What occurs directly after diffusion in the lungs?

A. air moves into the alveolar sacs.

B. carbon dioxide is exhaled from the body.

C. gases are transported by blood into circulation.

D. cells pick up oxygen in exchange for carbon dioxide.

26. Which describes the correct order of structures in the upper respiratory tract?

A. Lungs, heart, capillaries

B. Trachea, bronchus, lungs

C. Alveoli, bronchioles, trachea

D. Nasal cavity, pharynx, larynx

27. As air rushes out of the lungs, the

A. rib cage shortens.

B. bronchioles shrink.

C. diaphragm relaxes.

D. lungs change shape.

28. What is found in the medullary cavity?

A. Soft tissue

B. Red marrow

C. Compact bone

D. Articular cartilage

29. What is the portion of the vertebral column that has 12 bones?

A. coccyx   C. thoracic

B. lumbar   D. sacral

30. What is the purpose of ossification?

A. Destroy bone

B. Replace bone

C. Remodel bone

D. Generate bone

31. In which of the following segments do both secretion and reabsorption occur?

A. Loop of Henle

B. Collecting duct

C. Bowman's capsule

D. Distal convoluted tubule

32. What is one side effect of aging as it relates to the urinary system?

A. Increased bladder elasticity

B. Weakened bladder muscles

C. Replaced nephrons in the kidneys

D. Improved signaling between ADH and the kidneys

33. Where does the citric acid cycle occur in a cell?

A. Nucleus

B. Ribosome

C. Cytoplasm

D. Mitochondrion

34. Why is hydrogen bonding with water important?

A. It contributes to water's low boiling point.

B. It prevents water from being a universal solvent.

C. It creates weak interactions among water molecules.

D. It allows water in its solid form to float on liquid water.

35. A researcher characterizes the amino acid chain and structure of a novel substance. What type of substance is the researcher studying?

A. Fat   C. Enzyme

B. DNA   D. Sucrose

36. What happens during anabolic metabolism?

   A. Energy is released.

   B. Energy is absorbed.

   C. Nutrients are recycled.

   D. Substances are broken down.

37. Which organelle contains photosynthetic molecules?

   A. Chloroplast   C. Nucleolus

   B. Lysosome   D. Ribosome

38. Which organelles work together to protect a plant cell from the external environment?

   A. Flagella and pili

   B. Cytoplasm and lysosome

   C. Cell wall and cell membrane

   D. Ribosome and Golgi apparatus

39. Which process is part of photosynthesis?

   A. Anaphase   C. Calvin cycle

   B. Glycolysis   D. Pyruvate oxidation

40. Binary fission is a method

   A. where one daughter cell is produced.

   B. required to produce reproductive cells.

   C. that represents a form of asexual reproduction.

   D. where two parent cells interact with each other.

41. Before a molecule of glucose can be run through the citric acid cycle, it must experience

   A. ATP production.

   B. NADH production.

   C. pyruvate oxidation.

   D. oxygen deprivation.

42. How many sets of different chromosomes do human cells have?

   A. 12   C. 46

   B. 23   D. 50

43. The physical appearance or _____ of an organism is determined by a set of alleles.

   A. genotype   C. transcription

   B. phenotype   D. translation

44. An RNA copy of a gene used as a blueprint for a protein is called the _____.

   A. mRNA   C. rRNA

   B. pre-mRNA   D. tRNA

45. What is the function of a centromere?

   A. To connect the two chromatids

   B. To keep the chromosome stable

   C. To act as a relay point for genetic information

   D. To transmit genetic codes between other chromosomes

46. Refer to the Periodic Table of Elements and select which statement is true about 1 mole of carbon monoxide (CO).

   A. It contains 2 molecules.

   B. It contains 28.0 molecules.

   C. It has a mass of 28.0 grams.

   D. It has a mass of 6.02×10^{23} grams.

47. Three different dispersants that are used to break up oil in water are evaluated for their effectiveness. Dispersant A has a concentration of 10m, dispersant B has a concentration of 7m, and dispersant C has a concentration of 3m. Each dispersant is separately poured into a solution of water and oil. The amount of time it takes each dispersant to disperse the oil is recorded. Which of the following statements describes the positive correlation observed in this study?

    A. Oil remains suspended in solution despite dispersant addition.

    B. As more dispersant is added to the water, more oil is dispersed.

    C. Dispersant C is the least effective at dispersing oil in the solution of water.

    D. When a high concentration of dispersant is added, less oil disperses in water.

48. Which of the following statements is true?

    A. A tin atom has 22 protons.

    B. An iron atom has 26 protons.

    C. A sodium atom has 16 protons.

    D. A potassium atom has 15 protons.

49. How many electrons does a neutral atom of iodine have?

    A. 53   C. 126

    B. 74   D. 127

50. In the periodic table, which element is in period 5 and group 4?

    A. Manganese   C. Vanadium

    B. Molybdenum   D. Zirconium

51. An atom has 28 protons, 32 neutrons, and 28 electrons. What is the name of this isotope?

    A. Nickel-32

    B. Nickel-60

    C. Germanium-56

    D. Germanium-60

52. Which of the following properties is independent of the amount of matter in a substance?

    A. Chemical   C. Intensive

    B. Extensive   D. Physical

53. _____ is the ability of water to be attracted to other substances.

    A. Adhesion   C. Density

    B. Cohesion   D. Polar

SECTION IV. ENGLISH AND LANGUAGE USAGE

You have 28 minutes to complete 28 questions.

1. **Which of the following is correct?**

    A. american civil liberties union

    B. American civil liberties union

    C. American civil liberties Union

    D. American Civil Liberties Union

2. **What is the sentence with the correct use of quotation marks?**

    A. JFK said, Ask not what your country can do for you; ask what you can do for your country.

    B. JFK said, 'Ask not what your country can do for you; ask what you can do for your country.'

    C. JFK said, "Ask not what your country can do for you; ask what you can do for your country."

    D. JFK said a person must not ask what the country can do for them, but what they can do for their country.

3. **What is the correct plural of shelf?**

    A. Shelf   C. Shelfes

    B. Shelfs   D. Shelves

4. **Which of the following parts of speech correctly identifies the words "fast" and "faster" in this sentence?**

    Like the Wind is a <u>fast</u> racehorse, but *On the Mark* is <u>faster</u>.

    A. Noun   C. Adjective

    B. Verb   D. Adverb

5. **Identify the nouns in the following sentence.**

    Marie Curie won the Nobel Prize in 1911.

    A. won, in, 1911

    B. won, Nobel Prize, 1911

    C. Marie Curie, won, Nobel Prize

    D. Marie Curie, Nobel Prize, 1911

6. **Which of the following verbs CANNOT correctly complete this sentence?**

    ____ coat is so warm!

    A. My   C. This

    B. Her   D. Hers

7. **Which is <u>not</u> a prepositional phrase?**

    A. On the bus

    B. Against the wall

    C. Oh no

    D. To him

8. **What tense are the underlined verbs in the following sentence?**

    We <u>read</u> a book and <u>wrote</u> a paper about it.

    A. Simple past   C. Simple present

    B. Past perfect   D. Present perfect

9. **Which of the following verbs correctly completes this sentence?**

    Dolphins and fish ____ in that large tank.

    A. swim   C. swims

    B. swum   D. swimming

10. **Which of the following subjects correctly agrees with the verb "is" in this sentence?**

Anyone who has skates <u>is</u> invited to join us.

A. Anyone   C. skates

B. who   D. us

11. **Which of the following words is NOT a correct third person singular verb form?**

A. Does   C. Wishes

B. Its   D. Catches

12. **How would you connect the following clauses?**

The trial must begin.

She shows up or not.

A. The trial must begin and she shows up or not.

B. The trial must begin which she shows up or not.

C. The trial must begin because she shows up or not.

D. The trial must begin whether she shows up or not.

13. **Identify the independent clause in the following sentence.**

The mother could not take her kids to school because it snowed all night.

A. The mother could not take her kids

B. It snowed all night

C. Because it snowed all night

D. The mother could not take her kids to school

14. **Which sentence combines all of the information using a parallel structure?**

New York City is exciting. New York City is full of different cultures. New York City has so much to offer.

A. New York City is exciting, diverse, and interesting.

B. New York City has a lot of excitement, diverse, and interesting.

C. New York City is exciting, has different cultures, and interesting.

D. New York city is full of excitement, having different cultures, and it has so much to offer.

15. **Which of the following options correctly fixes the run-on sentence below?**

Taking a foreign language class is important speaking another language allows us to connect with others in our world.

A. Taking a foreign language class is important, speaking another language allows us to connect with others in our world.

B. Taking a foreign language class is important. Speaking another language allows us to connect with others in our world.

C. Taking a foreign language class is important and speaking another language allows us to connect with others in our world.

D. Taking a foreign language class is important speaking. Another language allows us to connect with others in our world.

16. Which of the following is an example of a simple sentence?

    A. Calcium for bones.

    B. Calcium makes bones strong.

    C. Calcium is necessary it makes bones strong.

    D. Calcium is good for bones, so people need it.

17. Which of the following sentences uses the MOST informal language?

    A. Great, thanks.

    B. That is wonderful. Thank you.

    C. Great job. Thank you.

    D. I appreciate your hard work.

18. In which of the following situations would you use formal language?

    A. Buying a car

    B. Calling your aunt

    C. Going to a movie

    D. Hiking with friends

19. Which of the following context clues correctly helps you define the word "grave" in this sentence?

    It was a grave situation, and people's lives were in danger.

    A. "situation"   C. "lives"

    B. "people's"   D. "danger"

20. Which of the following is the meaning of "tumultuous" as used in this sentence?

    The two have a tumultuous marriage filled with many ups and downs.

    A. Stormy   C. Interesting

    B. Solid   D. Terrible

21. Which of the following context clues correctly helps you define the word "taunt" in this sentence?

    The students gathered around and began to taunt the new student, making fun of the way she dressed and how she talked.

    A. "gathered around"

    B. "new student"

    C. "making fun"

    D. "way she dressed"

22. Which of the following words in this sentence has more than one meaning?

    The flu has the ability to strike millions of people each year, and some do not survive.

    A. Ability   C. Year

    B. Strike   D. Survive

23. Which of the following is the meaning of "confiscate" as used in this sentence?

    The school has a policy to confiscate all student cell phones before an exam so they are unable to cheat.

    A. Seize   C. Protect

    B. Hide   D. Store

24. Which of the following prefixes means "large"?

    A. con-   C. macro-

    B. rupt-   D. micro-

25. The use of the prefix *peri-* in the word periscope indicates which of the following about a person's view?

    A. She can see all around.

    B. She can see things behind her.

    C. She can only see things enlarged.

    D. She can only see heated things.

26. Something that is <u>amorphous</u> is

    A. toxic.   C. beneficial.

    B. shapeless.   D. enormous.

27. **Which of the following is the meaning of "quadruped" as used in this sentence?**

    A horse or a cow is an example of a <u>quadruped</u>.

    A. An animal that has fur

    B. An animal that is a mammal

    C. An animal that helps man

    D. An animal that has four feet

28. **Which of the following suffixes means "inflammation of"?**

    A. -itis   C. -ment

    B. -mort   D. -olgoy

TEAS Practice Exam 4
Answer Key with Explanatory Answers

Section I. Reading

1. C. The author of the paragraph begins and ends with an emphasis on the audience's enjoyment of disaster. This suggests that the main point has to do with the odd fact that people love disaster films. **Skill: Main Ideas, Topic Sentences, and Supporting Details.**

2. B. The final sentence sums up the main idea. This makes it the topic sentence. **Skill: Main Ideas, Topic Sentences, and Supporting Details.**

3. D. The author of this paragraph is making a point about how strange it is that people enjoy watching disasters unfold in fiction. By showing this happen before naming the phenomenon, the author maximizes the emotional impact. **Skill: Main Ideas, Topic Sentences, and Supporting Details.**

4. D. Supporting details should directly support the main idea of a text. Examples of violent forms of entertainment, and the enjoyment people take from them, could support the idea that people are naturally violent. **Skill: Main Ideas, Topic Sentences, and Supporting Details.**

5. C. If an author wanted to claim that disaster movies serve society in a positive way, he or she should emphasize the good qualities—like bravery and generosity—in these films. **Skill: Main Ideas, Topic Sentences, and Supporting Details.**

6. D. The pie chart indicates the amount of time students of different genders contribute to discussions. The larger wedge for male speaking indicates that 70% of class discussion time is dominated by male speakers. **Skill: Summarizing Text and Using Text Features.**

7. B. If you read the labels carefully, you will see that the bar graph shows how many times students of each gender *are interrupted* during class discussions. The graph shows that female students are interrupted more often than male students. **Skill: Summarizing Text and Using Text Features.**

8. B. The data in the chart and graph could help show that male students are receiving more chances to speak in class discussions, and that it would be a good idea to increase gender parity. **Skill: Summarizing Text and Using Text Features.**

9. B. To imply something is to suggest it rather than stating it explicitly. **Skill: Main Ideas, Topic Sentences, and Supporting Details.**

10. B. There is only one arrow leading from the start box, and it goes to the "look in the kitchen" box. **Skill: Summarizing Text and Using Text Features.**

11. D. The arrow that is labeled "No" directs readers to "Look in the kitchen." **Skill: Summarizing Text and Using Text Features.**

12. C. Graphic elements in a text present information visually in order to back up an argument, illustrate factual information or instructions, or present key facts and statistics. **Skill: Summarizing Text and Using Text Features.**

13. C. A summary may restate implicit ideas as long as they are clearly indicated in the original text. **Skill: Summarizing Text and Using Text Features.**

14. B. A pie chart shows percentages of a whole, so it would be a good option for showing how the economy is broken down into sectors. **Skill: Summarizing Text and Using Text Features.**

15. B. Quotations need to be properly introduced, explained, and cited. They do not need to be restated in different words because the content is there for the reader to see. **Skill: The Writing Process.**

16. C. A paragraph about the financial crisis and its consequences in the job market describes a cause and its effects. **Skill: The Writing Process.**

17. A. The first goal of writing is to be understood. Choose the simplest word unless you have a strong reason to do otherwise. **Skill: Essay Revision and Transitions.**

18. C. A transition is a connecting word or phrase that promotes smooth reading. **Skill: Essay Revision and Transitions.**

19. D. The second sentence expresses an idea that contrasts with the first. Therefore, the best transition is *nevertheless.* **Skill: Essay Revision and Transitions.**

20. C. A transition between these two sentences would likely suggest causation. Good choices would be words like *as a result* or *consequently.* **Skill: Tone, Mood, and Transition Words.**

21. C. This passage is a humorous description of a toddler's emotions, written by an adult who has enough experience to know that a toddler's huge emotions will pass. **Skill: Tone, Mood, and Transition Words.**

22. B. Authors use irony when their words do not literally mean what they say. The joy does not really go out of the world when a toddler loses her binky—but it may seem that way to the child. **Skill: Tone, Mood, and Transition Words.**

23. B. This passage establishes irony in the opening sentence by applying the superlative phrase "the most amazing thing ever" to an ordinary occurrence. **Skill: Tone, Mood, and Transition Words.**

24. A. Effective readers would likely know that this toddler's fear is nothing to worry about. Amusement would be a more likely reaction. **Skill: Tone, Mood, and Transition Words.**

25. B. The word "below" in paragraph one provides information about where the train is situated in relation to the character. It does not transition between ideas. **Skill: Tone, Mood, and Transition Words.**

26. A. "Later" and "afterward" are both time/sequence transitions that show when events happen in relation to one another. **Skill: Tone, Mood, and Transition Words.**

27. D. The author's point of view is his or her general outlook or set of opinions about the subject. **Skill: Understanding Author's Purpose, Point of View, and Rhetorical Strategies.**

28. B. Informational texts like cookbooks are usually meant to inform. **Skill: Understanding Author's Purpose, Point of View, and Rhetorical Strategies.**

29. B. Although the authors of this passage would likely agree with the argument that we need to address unconscious bias in our communities, the passage does not actually make such an argument. It only relays the survey results, words, and reported feelings of minority students on majority-white college campuses. **Skill: Understanding the Author's Purpose, Point of View, and Rhetorical Strategies.**

30. B. The authors of the passage are likely concerned with unconscious bias on college campuses and convinced that it has negative consequences, for example on job opportunities and future income. **Skill: Understanding the Author's Purpose, Point of View, and Rhetorical Strategies.**

31. A. The passage does not suggest that unconscious marginalization is the only force for racism in American society, and it certainly does not suggest that minority students need to learn to deal with racism better. However, it does suggest that unconscious bias is a problem that needs to be addressed. **Skill: Understanding the Author's Purpose, Point of View, and Rhetorical Strategies.**

32. B. The passage reports on the results of a survey and accompanying interviews. The quotations from the interviews add an emotional appeal by putting a human face on dry statistics. **Skill: Understanding the Author's Purpose, Point of View, and Rhetorical Strategies.**

33. A. The statistic shows that the majority of minority students felt marginalized on campus. **Skill: Understanding the Author's Purpose, Point of View, and Rhetorical Strategies.**

34. C. The main point of this paragraph is that science fiction often depicts a particular kind of post-apocalyptic survival scenario that would not work in fact. The title of the passage should reflect this idea. **Skill: Evaluating and Integrating Data.**

35. C. The author argues that the New York City subway system would not be a good place to take refuge after a major weather event if nobody were working to pump the water out. Information about the water would help illustrate that point. **Skill: Evaluating and Integrating Data.**

36. C. Sidebar information should be peripheral to the text. That means it's clearly related and interesting to the same audience. Here, the list of sci-fi novels would be the best option. **Skill: Evaluating and Integrating Data.**

37. C. Although the title of a fictional work may hint at a theme, a theme is a message that is, by definition, not stated explicitly. **Skill: Evaluating and Integrating Data.**

38. A. By convention, north on a map is up. Mapmakers include a compass if they break this convention for some reason. **Skill: Evaluating and Integrating Data.**

39. A. Biases may be stated or unstated, and they are not necessarily sweeping. They are preconceived and sometimes unfair ideas about the world. **Skill: Facts, Opinions, and Evaluating an Argument**

40. B. A stereotype is a particularly harmful kind of bias against a group of people. **Skill: Facts, Opinions, and Evaluating an Argument**

41. D. An opinion statement includes feelings or beliefs that are not necessarily verifiably true, but it may be based on valid reasoning. **Skill: Facts, Opinions, and Evaluating an Argument.**

42. C. Writers display gender bias when they use like *mankind* instead of *humankind* and when they write as if all people are male. **Skill: Facts, Opinions, and Evaluating an Argument.**

43. B. Writers show bias when they assume people of certain professions belong to certain genders. It is possible to write around this problem by using a plural. **Skill: Facts, Opinions, and Evaluating an Argument.**

44. C. Writers can eliminate gender bias by replacing a pronoun with *one, he,* or *she,* or an article (*a, an, the*). **Skill: Facts, Opinions, and Evaluating an Argument.**

45. A. Readers must use judgment to determine how credible a source is in a particular circumstance. An op-ed piece in a newspaper would be biased since it expresses the opinion of the author. **Skill: Understanding Primary Sources, Making Inferences, and Drawing Conclusions.**

46. D. Highly edited videos can be biased because parts could be purposely removed. **Skill: Understanding Primary Sources, Making Inferences, and Drawing Conclusions.**

47. A. From phrases like "your children," you can infer that the intended audience of this passage is parents. **Skill: Understanding Primary Sources, Making Inferences, and Drawing Conclusions.**

48. A. The author assumes that many parents have the problem of their children not listening to them or being able to focus well. **Skill: Understanding Primary Sources, Making Inferences, and Drawing Conclusions.**

49. C. The author does not suggest parents do not know how to discipline their children. This article is about setting limits on technology. It is not about disciplining children. **Skill: Understanding Primary Sources, Making Inferences, and Drawing Conclusions.**

50. B. Highly emotional arguments may be biased. In many cases, they make a source less credible. **Skill: Understanding Primary Sources, Making Inferences, and Drawing Conclusions.**

51. D. The structure of a text is its organizational scheme, not its category. Of the options above, a compare/contrast structure is most likely. **Skill: Types of Passages, Text Structures, Genre and Theme.**

52. C. An op-ed article argues a point, so it is a persuasive text. **Skill: Types of Passages, Text Structures, Genre and Theme.**

53. B. All of literature can be arranged into two basic categories, or genres: fiction and nonfiction. **Skill: Types of Passages, Text Structures, Genre and Theme.**

Section II. Mathematics

1. B. The correct solution is the team scored more than 65 points in a majority of games and gave up fewer than 65 points in a majority of games. From the graph, there are 6 games during which the team scored more than 65 points and 6 games during which it gave up fewer than 65 points. **Skill: Interpreting Graphics.**

2. C. The correct answer is $\frac{5}{6}$ because $\frac{15}{10} - \frac{2}{3} = \frac{45}{30} - \frac{20}{30} = \frac{25}{30} = \frac{5}{6}$. **Skill: Addition and Subtraction of Fractions.**

3. C. There are 300 cattle in the herd. Because the herd is only Ayrshire or Jersey, it is 65% Jersey. The equivalent decimals are 0.35 Ayrshire and 0.65 Jersey. Set up a proportion that relates these decimals to the number of cattle of each type:

$$\frac{0.35}{0.65} = \frac{?}{195}$$

One approach is to divide 195 by 0.65 to get 300, then multiply by 0.35 to get the number of Ayrshires: 105. Add 195 and 105 to get the total number of cattle in the herd. **Skill: Ratios, Proportions, and Percentages.**

4. C. Ratios act just like fractions, so this product is the product of $\frac{3}{2}$ and $\frac{5}{6}$, or $\frac{15}{12} = \frac{5}{4}$. **Skill: Ratios, Proportions, and Percentages.**

5. C. The company employs 273 men. If 35% of the company's employees are women, 65% are men. Set up a proportion using 65%, which is equal to $\frac{65}{100}$ or $\frac{13}{20}$:

$$\frac{13}{20} = \frac{?}{420}$$

The unknown number is the product of 13 and 420 ÷ 20 = 21, which is 273. **Skill: Ratios, Proportions, and Percentages.**

6. B. The correct solution is 50. The middle two values are 40 and 60, and the average of these values is 50. **Skill: Interpreting Categorical and Quantitative Data.**

7. A. It will take Henry 36 minutes to get home because $\frac{50\ miles}{60\ minutes} = \frac{30\ miles}{36\ minutes}$. **Skill: Solving Real World Mathematical Problems.**

8. D. The correct solution is 60.98 centimeters. $2\ ft \times \frac{1\ m}{3.28\ ft} \times \frac{100\ cm}{1\ m} = \frac{200}{3.28} = 60.98\ cm$. **Skill: Standards of Measure.**

9. D. Converting answers A and D to decimals yields (approximately) 0.44 and 2.25, respectively. Answers B and C are both equal to 0.44, so answer D differs from the others. **Skill: Ratios, Proportions, and Percentages.**

10. B. The correct solution is $x–xy–2y$.

$$(8x + 2xy–4y) + (–7x–3xy + 2y) = (8x–7x) + (2xy–3xy) + (–4y + 2y) = x–xy–2y$$

Skill: Polynomials.

11. A. The correct answer is 1.455 because 145.5% as a decimal is 145.5 ÷ 100 = 1.455. **Skill: Decimals and Fractions.**

12. D. Using the appropriate conversion equation, $(75°F – 32) \times \frac{5}{9} = 23.88$ or 24°C. **Skill: Standards of Measure.**

13. D. Alan paid $37, 296 for the car in total because $518 x 12 months in a year = $6,216 a year x 6 years = $37, 296. **Skill: Solving Real World Mathematical Problems.**

14. A. The correct solution is A because the points for each city are graphed correctly. **Skill: Interpreting Graphics.**

15. B. The correct answer is $0.8\overline{3}$ because $83.\overline{3}\%$ as a decimal is $0.8\overline{3}$. **Skill: Decimals and Fractions.**

16. B. The correct solution is 500,000 milliliters. $0.5\ kL \times \frac{1,000\ L}{1\ kL} \times \frac{1,000\ mL}{1\ L} = 500,000\ mL$. **Skill: Standards of Measure.**

17. C. Hannah earns $36,550 because there are 52 weeks in a year because 365 ÷ 7 ≈ 52. After subtracting out 1 week of the year for unpaid time off, Hannah is paid 17 paychecks because 51 ÷ 3 = 17. Multiplying 17 by her salary of $2150 a paycheck, she earns $36,550 annually. **Skill: Solving Real World Mathematical Problems.**

18. A. The correct solution is classes F, G, and H collected more than 150 items. Class F collected 160 items, class G collected 180 items, and class H collected 170 items. **Skill: Interpreting Graphics.**

19. D. The correct solution is 28 because $x^2 = 81 + 3 = 84 \div 3 = 28$. **Skill: Equations with One Variable.**

20. B. The correct solution is $4\frac{13}{16}$ because $\frac{11}{2} \times \frac{7}{8} = \frac{77}{16} = 4\frac{13}{16}$. **Skill: Multiplication and Division of Fractions.**

21. D. The correct solution is $3\frac{1}{2}$ because $\frac{3}{2} \times \frac{7}{3} = \frac{21}{6} = 3\frac{3}{6} = 3\frac{1}{2}$. **Skill: Multiplication and Division of Fractions.**

22. B. The correct solution is $\frac{25}{17}$.

$9(x + 3) - 24 = 36 - 8(x + 1)$	Multiply all terms by the least common denominator of 12 to eliminate the fractions.
$9x + 27 - 24 = 36 - 8x - 8$	Apply the distributive property.
$9x + 3 = 28 - 8x$	Combine like terms on both sides of the equation.
$17x + 3 = 28$	Add $8x$ to both sides of the equation.
$17x = 25$	Subtract 3 from both sides of the equation.
$x = \frac{25}{17}$	Divide both sides of the equation by 17.

Skill: Equations with One Variable.

23. C. The correct answer is $77.\overline{7}\%$ because $\frac{7}{9}$ as a percent is $\frac{7}{9} = 0.\overline{7} \times 100 = 77.\overline{7}\%$. **Skill: Decimals and Fractions.**

24. A. The correct solution is 8 because the equation simplifies to 2x = 16 and x = 8. **Skill: Equations with One Variable.**

25. B. The correct solution is 16. Substitute the values into the formula $448 = 2l(14)$ and simplify the right side of the equation, $448 = 28l$. Divide both sides of the equation by 28, $l = 16$ feet. **Skill: Similarity, Right Triangles, and Trigonometry.**

26. A. The correct solution is $\frac{1}{10}$ because $1 - \left(\frac{1}{6} + \frac{2}{5} + \frac{1}{3}\right) = 1 - \left(\frac{5}{30} + \frac{12}{30} + \frac{10}{30}\right) = 1 - \frac{27}{30} = 1 - \frac{9}{10} = \frac{1}{10}$ of the yard remaining. **Skill: Solving Real World Mathematical Problems.**

27. D. It costs an extra $1,800 a year to have a second bedroom because the difference per month is $150 x 12 = $1,800 a year. **Skill: Solving Real World Mathematical Problems.**

28. C. The correct solution is 4. Substitute the values into the formula, $400 = 2l(8) + 2l(14) + 2(8)(14)$, and simplify using order of operations, $400 = 16l + 28l + 224; 400 = 44l + 224$. Then, subtract 224 from both sides of the equation and divide both sides of the equation by 44, $176 = 44l$; $l = 4$ inches. **Skill: Similarity, Right Triangles, and Trigonometry.**

29. A. The correct solution is −8.

$\frac{x}{4} = -2$	Subtract 8 from both sides of the equation.
$x = -8$	Multiply both sides of the equation by 4.

Skill: Equations with One Variable.

30. D. The correct solution is 60.64 liters. $16 \, gal \times \frac{3.79 \, L}{1 \, gal} = 60.64 \, L$. **Skill: Standards of Measure.**

31. B. The correct solution is 11.5 centimeters because $C = 2\pi r; 72 = (2)3.14r; 72 = 6.28r; r \approx 11.5$ centimeters. **Skill: Circles.**

32. C. The correct solution is C because each of the percent values is calculated correctly. There are 15 parts for the mix. The percents for eggs and oil are each $\frac{2}{15} = 0.1333 = 13.33\%$. The percent for water is $\frac{3}{15} = \frac{1}{5} = 0.20 = 20\%$. The percent for mixture is $\frac{7}{15} = 0.4667 = 46.67\%$. The percent for vanilla is $\frac{1}{15} = 0.0667 = 6.67\%$. **Skill: Interpreting Graphics.**

33. B. The correct response is B. The median value is 12.5, the first quartile value is 8, and the third quartile value is 17. The minimum is 5, and the maximum is 20. **Skill: Interpreting Categorical and Quantitative Data.**

34. C. The correct solution is 3,375. Substitute the values into the formula and simplify using the order of operations, $V = s^3 = 15^3 = 3,375$ cubic millimeters. **Skill: Similarity, Right Triangles, and Trigonometry.**

35. D. The correct solution is $y = \frac{C-Ax}{B}$.

$By = C-Ax$ Subtract Ax from both sides of the equation.

$y = \frac{C-Ax}{B}$ Divide both sides of the equation by B.

Skill: Equations with One Variable.

36. D. 1 gram is equal to 1,000 milligrams, so the nurse is providing 500 milligrams of medicine with each dose. $2500 \div 500 = 5$ doses. **Skill: Solving Real World Mathematical Problems.**

Section III. Science

1. B. The chemical level of organization involves interactions among atoms and their combinations into molecules. **Skill: Organization of the Human Body.**

2. B. The term *deep* means "away from the surface." **Skill: Organization of the Human Body.**

3. A. *Dorsal* is synonymous with *posterior* and means "toward the back." **Skill: Organization of the Human Body.**

4. D. A vascular spasm or vasoconstriction occurs first during wound healing. Then, a platelet plug forms, followed by blood coagulation. After a fibrin mesh is formed during coagulation, the wounded site is closed. **Skill: Cardiovascular System.**

5. D. Blood is composed of liquid plasma, a buffy coat, and a reddish mass. Found at the bottom of a spun-down blood sample, the reddish mass containing erythrocytes is the densest component of blood. **Skill: Cardiovascular System.**

6. A. Autocrine chemical signals are released by cells and have a local effect on the same cell type. **Skill: Endocrine System.**

7. D. Monosaccharides are the foundational units of carbohydrates. **Skill: Gastrointestinal System.**

8. A. Amylase is secreted in the mouth, and it is the first enzyme that goes into action. **Skill: Gastrointestinal System.**

9. A. The gallbladder is nestled under the liver and stores the bile the liver makes. **Skill: Gastrointestinal System.**

10. C. The cecum is a blind pouch where the small intestine meets the large intestine. **Skill: Gastrointestinal System.**

11. C. The nail plate is the outer part of the nail that protects the edges of the finger. This structure is hard and connected to the free edge of the nail. **Skill: Integumentary System.**

12. A. Atrial systole occurs when the atrium contracts. On an EKG, atrial systole is indicated by a P wave. **Skill: Cardiovascular System.**

13. B. Neuroglia are cells that support neurons in the body. More neuroglia are present in the body than neurons. Four types are found in the CNS, and two types are found in the PNS. **Skill: The Nervous System.**

14. D. The axial skeleton consists of bones that do not belong to the upper and lower extremities: the skull, vertebral column, sternum, and ribcage. **Skill: The Skeletal System.**

15. B. As people age, their bodies produce fewer B and T cells. As a result, the body's ability to defend itself against viruses and bacteria lessens. **Skill: The Lymphatic System.**

16. B. There are two kidneys in the body, which are located below the rib cage. The kidneys filter the blood that comes from the heart and remove wastes from the blood. **Skill: The Urinary System.**

17. D. The A-band is dark band that consists of thick and thin, or myosin and actin, filaments. Arrangements of myosin and actin myofilaments create this band. **Skill: Muscular System.**

18. C. Fibrous joints are also known as immovable joints. They are a type of connective tissue that joins bones that are in close contact with each other. **Skill: Muscular System.**

19. B. There are four primary functions of the muscular system: provide support, stabilize joints, generate heat, and aid in body movement. Through muscle contraction and relaxation, muscles generate heat for the body. **Skill: Muscular System.**

20. C. A neural impulse transmits electric signals down the axon of a neuron to the axon terminal. Following the stimulation of a neural impulse, an action potential is established, which triggers the synaptic transmission process between two neurons. **Skill: The Nervous System.**

21. D. After calcium ions flood into the axon bulb, it triggers the synaptic vesicle to contract and move closer to the presynaptic membrane of the neuron. Once close enough, it fuses to the membrane and undergoes exocytosis, releasing neurotransmitters into the synaptic cleft. The neurotransmitters diffuse across this cleft and bind to receptors. **Skill: The Nervous System.**

22. A. The synaptic cleft is the region between a pre- and postsynaptic membrane. This is the site across which neurotransmitters diffuse to bind to receptors on the postsynaptic membrane of a neuron, muscle cell, or gland. **Skill: The Nervous System.**

23. C. If the ovum is not fertilized, it passes out of the body with the menstrual flow. **Skill: Reproductive System.**

24. C. Nutrients leave the mother through the uterine wall of the uterus, passing first into the placenta and then along the umbilical to the fetus. Fetal waste follows the reverse course. **Skill: Reproductive System.**

25. C. During external respiration, air is first inhaled into the lungs via pulmonary ventilation. Then, diffusion of oxygen from the lungs into the blood occurs. Next, oxygenated blood is transported through systemic circulation. **Skill: The Respiratory System.**

26. D. Within the upper respiratory tract, air enters the body through the nasal cavity. Next, it proceeds to the pharynx and larynx. **Skill: The Respiratory System.**

27. C. As air rushes out of the lungs, the diaphragm relaxes and returns to its characteristic dome shape. This allows the rib cage to return to its position. **Skill: The Respiratory System.**

28. B. The medullary cavity is a hollow opening inside the long bone. It consists of red and yellow bone marrow. **Skill: Skeletal System.**

29. C. The vertebral column contains 24 bones called the pre-sacral vertebrae. Twelve of these bones belong to the thoracic region. In addition to these 24 bones, there is the sacrum and coccyx. There is a total of 26 bones of the vertebral column. **Skill: Skeletal System.**

30. D. Ossification is the process of bone formation. It is used during fetal development to transform cartilage into mineralized hard bone tissue. **Skill: Skeletal System.**

31. D. Tubular reabsorption involves a process during which the filtered fluid contains solutes and water that are reabsorbed into the bloodstream. Nitrogenous wastes are secreted in the distal convoluted tubule to be excreted from the body. **Skill: The Urinary System.**

32. B. As the body ages, so do the bladder and kidneys. Nephron loss occurs, and the bladder loses its elasticity. When this decreased elasticity is coupled with weakened bladder muscles, a person may have trouble urinating voluntarily. **Skill: The Urinary System.**

33. D. Glycolysis is the only metabolic pathway that takes place in the cytoplasm of a cell. The citric acid cycle, electron transport chain, and oxidative phosphorylation take place in the cell's mitochondria. **Skill: An Introduction to Biology.**

34. C. Hydrogen bonding is a type of weak attraction that forms between water molecules. **Skill: An Introduction to Biology.**

35. C. Amino acids are the monomers used to make proteins. An example of a protein is an enzyme. **Skill: An Introduction to Biology.**

36. B. During anabolic metabolism, energy is absorbed as new substances like polymers are created. **Skill: An Introduction to Biology.**

37. A. Chloroplasts are organelles that trap energy from the sun and use this to help plants create food. They contain chlorophyll molecules, which are photosynthetic pigments. **Skill: Cell Structure, Function, and Type.**

38. C. The cell wall provides structural support and protects the cell from the external environment. The cell membrane is selectively permeable, allowing only certain things from the outside environment to enter. **Skill: Cell Structure, Function, and Type.**

39. C. Photosynthesis consists of light reactions and dark reactions. The dark reactions are referred to as the Calvin cycle. **Skill: Cellular Reproduction, Cellular Respiration, and Photosynthesis.**

40. C. Binary fission is a method organisms use to reproduce asexually. It involves a single parent cell that splits to create two identical daughter cells. **Skill: Cellular Reproduction, Cellular Respiration, and Photosynthesis.**

41. C. A glucose molecule must first experience pyruvate oxidation because one CO_2 molecule must be removed from each pyruvate molecule after glycolysis and before the citric acid cycle. **Skill: Cellular Reproduction, Cellular Respiration, and Photosynthesis.**

42. B. Humans have 23 sets of chromosomes. **Skill: Genetics and DNA.**

43. B. The phenotype is the physical appearance of an organism, and the genotype is the set of alleles. **Skill: Genetics and DNA.**

44. A. A copy of a gene used as a blueprint for a protein is mRNA. **Skill: Genetics and DNA.**

45. A. The protein disc that connects the two chromatids is the centromere. **Skill: Genetics and DNA.**

46. C. A mole of CO contains 6.02×10^{23} molecules and has a mass of 28.0 g/mol. The molar mass was calculated by adding the molar mass of carbon (12.0 g/mol) to the molar mass of oxygen (16.0 g/mol). **Skill: Chemical Equations.**

47. B. A positive correlation means that one variable increases as another increases. Thus, as more dispersant is added, the amount of oil dispersed also increases. **Skill: Designing an Experiment.**

48. B. In the periodic table, iron has an atomic number of 26, which means it has 26 protons. **Skill: Scientific Notation.**

49. A. In a neutral atom, the number of electrons is equal to the number of protons. Because the atomic number of iodine is 53, there are 53 protons and 53 electrons to balance the charge. **Skill: Scientific Notation.**

50. D. To find this element, find the element in the fifth row (period) and the fourth column (group). **Skill: Scientific Notation.**

51. B. The number of protons, 28, gives the atomic number, which identifies this atom as nickel. The mass is the number after the dash in the isotope name, which is determined by adding the numbers of protons and neutrons (28 + 32 = 60). **Skill: Scientific Notation.**

52. C. Intensive properties do not change based on the amount of matter in a substance. **Skill: Properties of Matter.**

53. A. Adhesion is the ability of water to be attracted to other substances. **Skill: Properties of Matter.**

Section IV. English and Language Usage

1. D. American Civil Liberties Union. National organizations need to be capitalized. **Skill: Capitalization.**

2. C. *JFK said, "Ask not what your country can do for you; ask what you can do for your country."* Quotation marks enclose words or sentences that someone else said or wrote. **Skill: Punctuation.**

3. D. With words ending in -f, drop the -f and add -ves. **Skill: Spelling.**

4. C. These words are adjectives that describe the noun *racehorse*. **Skill: Adjectives and Adverbs.**

5. D. *Marie Curie, Nobel Prize*, and *1911* are nouns. **Skill: Nouns.**

6. D. *Hers* cannot be used to modify a noun. **Skill: Pronouns.**

7. C. *Oh no* is an interjection. It does not contain a preposition. **Skill: Conjunctions and Prepositions.**

8. A. *Read* and *wrote* are in simple past tense. **Skill: Verbs and Verb Tenses.**

9. A. *Dolphins and fish* is a third person plural subject, so it takes the verb form *swim*. **Skill: Subject and Verb Agreement.**

10. A. The verb *is* agrees with the subject *anyone. Who has skates* is a relative clause; it is not the main subject. **Skill: Subject and Verb Agreement.**

11. B. The word *its* is the possessive for *it*. It is not a verb. **Skill: Subject and Verb Agreement.**

12. D. The trial must begin whether she shows up or not. With an independent and dependent clause, a subordinating conjunction is used to connect them. "Whether" is the only choice that makes sense. **Skill: Types of Clauses.**

13. D. The mother could not take her kids to school. It is independent because it has a subject, verb, and expresses a complete thought. **Skill: Types of Clauses.**

14. A. This sentence combines the information using parallel structure. **Skill: Types of Sentences.**

15. B. This sentence correctly fixes the run-on sentence. **Skill: Types of Sentences.**

16. B. This is a simple sentence since it contains one independent clause consisting of a simple subject and a predicate. **Skill: Types of Sentences.**

17. A. Great, thanks. The sentence is the most informal as it uses slang. **Skill: Formal and Informal Language.**

18. A. Buying a car. It is best to use formal language with the car salesperson as he or she is probably not a close acquaintance. **Skill: Formal and Informal Language.**

19. D. The meaning of grave in this context is "very serious." The phrase "danger" helps you figure out which meaning of grave is being used. **Skill: Context Clues and Multiple Meaning Words.**

20. A. The meaning of tumultuous in the context of this sentence is "stormy." **Skill: Context Clues and Multiple Meaning Words.**

21. C. The meaning of taunt in this context is "to say insulting things to." The phrase "making fun" helps you figure out the meaning of taunt. **Skill: Context Clues and Multiple Meaning Words.**

22. B. The word "strike" has more than one meaning. **Skill: Context Clues and Multiple Meaning Words.**

23. A. The meaning of confiscate in the context of this sentence is "seize." **Skill: Context Clues and Multiple Meaning Words.**

24. C. The prefix that means "large" is *macro-* as in the word *macroeconomics*. **Skill: Root Words, Prefixes, and Suffixes.**

25. A. The prefix *peri-* means "around," and the root word *scope* means "to watch and see," so a periscope would enable a person to see all around. **Skill: Root Words, Prefixes, and Suffixes.**

26. B. The root *morph* means "form," and the prefix *a-* means "without or not," so something that is amorphous is shapeless. **Skill: Root Words, Prefixes, and Suffixes.**

27. D. The prefix *quad-* means "four," and the root word *ped* means "foot," so a quadruped is an animal that has four feet. **Skill: Root Words, Prefixes, and Suffixes.**

28. A. The suffix that means "inflammation of" is *-itis* as in the word *tonsillitis*. **Skill: Root Words, Prefixes, and Suffixes.**

TEAS PRACTICE EXAM 5

SECTION I. READING

You have 64 minutes to complete 53 questions.

Please read the text below and answer questions 1-3.

It is perhaps unsurprising that school dress codes are becoming more common in American public schools. In our high-status-driven society, students feel the pressure to keep up with the most current fashion trends. The additional anxiety of wanting to "fit in" with peers can distract students from performing their best academically. In addition, some fashion trends are downright inappropriate and can be distracting to other students! Enforcing a dress code can allow schools to offer guidelines for clothing options that are suitable for school. Some school administrators are in favor of requiring students to wear a specific school uniform. Others suggest this may not be the most advantageous option as cost could still be a factor for some students, resulting in the same level of anxiety. Instead, they argue, offering simple guidelines that afford students the ability to meet their school's dress code requirements with maximum flexibility.

1. **The topic of this paragraph is:**

   A. fashion trends.

   B. dress codes.

   C. school uniforms.

   D. academic excellence.

2. **The topic sentence of this paragraph is:**

   A. In our high-status-driven society, students feel the pressure to keep up with the most current fashion trends.

   B. Enforcing a dress code can allow schools to offer guidelines for clothing options that are suitable for school

   C. Some school administrators are in favor of requiring students to wear specific a school uniform.

   D. Others suggest this may not be the most advantageous option as cost could still be a factor for some students, resulting in the same level of anxiety.

3. **If the author added a description of a student who wore inappropriate outfits to school and ended up distracting other students, what type of information would this be?**

   A. A main idea

   B. A topic sentence

   C. A supporting detail

   D. An off-topic sentence

4. **Which graphic would you use to show a sequence of decisions involved in a complex process?**

   A. Diagram

   B. Flowchart

   C. Bar graph

   D. Pie chart

5. Which graphic would you use to convey the differences between numerical values using rectangles?

   A. Diagram
   C. Bar graph
   B. Flowchart
   D. Pie chart

6. What must every body paragraph do?

   A. Introduce the topic
   B. Ask a compelling question
   C. Follow chronological order
   D. Relate clearly to the main point

7. What type of paragraph hooks the reader's interest, provides background information on the topic, and states the main point?

   A. Body paragraph
   B. Sequential paragraph
   C. Introductory paragraph
   D. Cause/effect paragraph

8. Which structure would most likely fit a paragraph describing the reasons why the SmartMouth 2000 electric toothbrush is better than its competitors?

   A. Sequential
   C. Cause/effect
   B. Descriptive
   D. Compare/contrast

9. Which of the following is a way of organizing ideas?

   A. Outlining
   B. Free writing
   C. Brainstorming
   D. Conducting research

Read the following sentence and answer questions 10-11.

The _____ of her perfume lingered in the air long after she left.

10. Which word, if inserted into the space above, would clearly establish a positive tone?

    A. reek
    C. stench
    B. smell
    D. fragrance

11. Which word, if inserted into the space above, would clearly establish a negative tone?

    A. smell
    C. aroma
    B. stench
    D. fragrance

12. Read the following sentence:

    Studies of chimpanzee behavior suggest that the preoccupation with jealousy and fairness is not unique to man.

    Which revision gives the sentence greater inclusivity?

    A. A Rice University study of chimpanzee behavior suggests that the preoccupation with jealousy and fairness is not unique to man.

    B. A Rice University study of chimpanzee behavior suggest that the preoccupation with jealousy and fairness is not unique to mankind.

    C. Studies of chimpanzee behavior suggest that the preoccupation with jealousy and fairness is not unique to human beings.

    D. No change.

13. Read the following sentence:

Her neighbors don't get why she took out that tree.

Which word choice revision would make the sentence more formal without changing the meaning?

A. Her neighbors do not understand why she removed that tree.

B. Her neighbors do not receive compensation for the tree she removed.

C. The people who live near her do not get why she chopped down that tree.

D. Her neighbors don't get what her reasons were for destroying her shrubberies.

14. **What is *not* a quality of rhetorically effective writing?**

A. It inspires the reader's trust.

B. It avoids all gendered pronouns.

C. It is grounded in logic and reasoning.

D. It engages the emotions appropriately.

15. **Read the sentences below.**

Jose is a determined individual. _____ he spent five days trying to teach himself the guitar since he wants to join a band. _____ his mom claims that he exhibited similar behavior when he wanted to walk; he spent hours getting up and falling down.

Which words or phrases should be inserted into the blanks to provide clear transitions between these ideas?

A. In conclusion; Thus

B. First; Consequently

C. Although; In contrast

D. For instance; Moreover

16. **Which word functions as a transition in the sentence below?**

Cassandra loved reading and writing books as a child. Thus, she became an English teacher in her adult life.

A. Loved   C. Thus

B. Child   D. Became

17. **Which word functions as a transition in the sentences below?**

However you celebrate the holidays, it's time to spend with your family. It's also a time to enjoy some good food!

A. However   C. Also

B. Time   D. Some

18. **Which aspects of the text are most important in establishing mood?**

A. Setting and theme

B. Parallelism and syntax

C. Organization and structure

D. Transitions and conjunctions

19. **Tone and mood are similar concepts, but readers need both terms in order to discuss differences between:**

A. the author's attitude and the reader's reactions.

B. the words for feelings and the experience of emotion.

C. the author's feelings and the characters' personalities.

D. the reactions of two different readers of the same text.

20. **Which term describes a connecting word or phrase that helps readers follow the flow of a writer's thoughts?**

A. Transition   C. Connotation

B. Denotation   D. Juxtaposition

21. **Which of the following is *not* a common function of transitions?**

    A. Introducing an example

    B. Orienting the reader in time

    C. Telling the reader the mood

    D. Creating a sense of emphasis

22. **Read the sentences below.**

    Jeremiah's lacrosse season had a rocky start. He is determined to score more goals than his teammates this year.

    Which word or phrase, if inserted at the beginning of sentence two, would effectively transition between these two ideas?

    A. Likewise   C. For example

    B. Previously   D. Nevertheless

Read the passages below and answer questions 23-31.

Electroconvulsive therapy was pioneered in the 1930s as a method for combatting severe psychiatric symptoms such as intractable depression and paranoid schizophrenia. This procedure, which involves delivering a deliberate electrical shock to the brain, was controversial from the beginning because it caused pain and short-term memory loss. It fell strongly out of public favor after the 1962 publication of Ken Kesey's novel *One Flew Over the Cuckoo's Nest*, which featured an unprincipled nurse using electroconvulsive therapy as a means of control over her patients. Paradoxically, medical advances at the time of the novel's publication made electroconvulsive therapy significantly safer and more humane.

Although the public is still generally opposed to electroconvulsive therapy, it remains a genuine option for psychiatric patients whose symptoms do not improve with medication. Medical professionals who offer this option should be especially careful to make clear distinctions between myth and reality. On this topic, unfortunately, many patients tend to rely on fiction rather than fact.

*

We were led into a stark exam room, where three doctors positioned themselves so Mama and I had no direct path to the door. The one in charge cleared his throat and told me my mother needed electroshock. My brain buzzed—almost as if it was hooked up to some crackpot brainwashing machine—as Big Doctor droned on about his sadistic intentions. I didn't hear any of it. All I could think was that these people wanted to tie my mother down and stick wires in her ears.

When Big Doctor was finished, he flipped through the papers on his clipboard and asked if I had questions. I mumbled something noncommittal. Then, when he and his silent escort left, I grabbed Mama and beat it out of that wacko ward as fast as I could make her go.

23. **What is the purpose of the first paragraph of Passage 1?**

    A. To inform   C. To persuade

    B. To distract   D. To entertain

24. What is the purpose of the second paragraph of Passage 1?

    A. To inform   C. To persuade

    B. To distract   D. To entertain

25. What is the primary purpose of Passage 2?

    A. To inform   C. To persuade

    B. To distract   D. To entertain

26. With which statement would the author of Passage 1 likely agree?

    A. Patients who suffer from mental illness should sue Ken Kesey for libel.

    B. Electroconvulsive therapy is a ready solution for every psychiatric complaint.

    C. No twenty-first century patient should ever receive electroconvulsive therapy.

    D. Medical patients should try options such as medication before electroconvulsive therapy.

27. Which detail from Passage 1 supports the conclusion that patients should try other options before electing to undergo electroconvulsive therapy?

    A. This procedure...was controversial from the beginning because it caused pain and short-term memory loss.

    B. Ken Kesey's novel *One Flew Over the Cuckoo's Nest*...featured an unprincipled nurse using electroconvulsive therapy as a means of control over her patients.

    C. Electroconvulsive therapy...remains a genuine option for patients whose symptoms do not improve with medication.

    D. Paradoxically, medical advances at the time of the novel's publication made electroconvulsive therapy significantly safer and more humane.

28. The author of Passage 1 would most likely criticize the author of Passage 2 for:

    A. failing to listen to the doctor's explanations.

    B. making no attempt to protect her ailing mother.

    C. feeling threatened by her physical circumstances.

    D. asking too many questions and wasting the doctor's time.

29. The author of Passage 1 would most likely criticize the doctor in Passage 2 for:

A. revealing medical information to the patient's family members.

B. denying the patient and her family the chance to ask questions.

C. taking control of the meeting instead of letting underlings speak.

D. neglecting to anticipate the feelings of his patient and her family.

30. Which details from Passage 2 suggest that the author has a negative outlook about medical professionals?

A. She describes feeling trapped in a room by doctors, one of whom she calls "sadistic."

B. She describes feeling outnumbered when she makes reasoned arguments to a doctor she calls "wacko."

C. She describes feeling bored by the idea that the doctor wants to "tie [her] mother down and stick wires in her ears."

D. She describes feeling excited by the prospect of seeing her mother hooked up to a pseudo-medical "brainwashing machine."

31. The author of Passage 1 supports her points primarily by:

A. telling humanizing stories.

B. relying on facts and logic.

C. pointing to expert sources.

D. using fear tactics and manipulation.

32. The purpose of an index is to tell readers:

A. how to find sources that back up key ideas in the text.

B. who wrote the text and what his or her credentials are.

C. where to find information on a given subject within a book.

D. why the author believes the main idea of a text is important.

33. If you are researching a topic and want to know if a particular book contains information on it, which text feature is most likely to be useful to you?

A. Sidebars   C. Boldfacing

B. Footnotes   D. Table of contents

34. On a chart, horizontal lines are called _____, whereas vertical lines are called _____.

A. keys, rows   C. rows, columns

B. legends, keys   D. columns, legends

35. Grant is reading a map, and he sees a symbol he does not understand. What should he do?

A. Ask for directions.

B. Consult a compass.

C. Adjust the map's scale.

D. Look for a key or legend.

Read the following paragraphs and answer questions 36-42.

The idea of raising children in prison is controversial, but well-run prison nursery programs can actually be beneficial. A study of preschool age children showed that anxiety and depression are common among young children who are separated from their mothers at birth and reunited later. In contrast, babies who spent brief sentences of two years or less behind bars with their mothers showed greater resilience and stronger attachments.

According to a nationwide analysis of women who participated in prison nursery programs, the benefits for mothers are even clearer than the benefits to children. Women who were allowed to remain with their infants during prison sentences were less likely to be convicted of another crime and less likely to use drugs in the five years after release. They were more likely to continue their education in prison and more likely to find employment on the outside. Mothers involved in prison nursery programs also reported better mental health and greater confidence in their own parenting skills.

36. **Which statement expresses an opinion?**

    A. A study of preschool age children showed that anxiety and depression are common among young children who are separated from their mothers at birth and reunited later.

    B. The idea of raising children in prison is controversial, but well-run prison nursery programs can actually be beneficial.

    C. Mothers involved in prison nursery programs also reported better mental health and greater confidence in their own parenting skills.

    D. Women who were allowed to remain with their infants during prison sentences were less likely to be convicted of another crime and less likely to use drugs after release.

37. **Consider the following sentence from the passage:**

    Mothers involved in prison nursery programs also reported better mental health and greater confidence in their own parenting skills.

    Is this statement a fact or an opinion? Why?

    A. An opinion because it shares information about confidence, which is an emotion.

    B. A fact because it states verifiable information about how women reported they felt.

    C. A fact because it focuses on information from medical records rather than faulty memories.

    D. An opinion because it relies on human input rather than objective sources like computer records.

38. **What is the primary argument of the passage?**

    A. Young children should not be forced to live in prisons.

    B. Society must promote the health and safety of children.

    C. Letting imprisoned mothers keep their babies can be helpful.

    D. It is bad for children but good for mothers if children live in prison.

39. **What is one assumption behind the passage?**

    A. Imprisoned mothers should take parenting classes to learn how to raise children.

    B. Some people disagree with the idea of allowing mothers to raise children in prison.

    C. The needs of incarcerated mothers are more important than the needs of their babies.

    D. Society should protect the health and well-being of children born to incarcerated mothers.

40. **Which sentence responding to the passage displays faulty reasoning?**

    A. Although prison nursery programs have benefits, they do not justify the costs.

    B. Putting babies in jail is wrong because people that young do not belong in prison.

    C. Further research is necessary before it becomes a common practice to incarcerate babies.

    D. Society needs to find a better solution than prison for babies with incarcerated mothers.

41. **The paragraph in the passage about benefits to mothers contains faulty reasoning because it:**

    A. suggests a cause-and-effect relationship without proving it.

    B. causes readers to question the mothers' mental health outcomes.

    C. does not prove factually that women in the program are better mothers.

    D. fails to show that it is beneficial to participate in prison education programs.

42. **Read the following sentences:**

    We must provide funding to expand prison nursery programs to serve all women who give birth in prison. To do otherwise would cause babies to suffer needlessly.

    This would be an *ineffective* conclusion to the passage above because:

    A. it uses circular reasoning.

    B. it uses either/or reasoning.

    C. its language includes insults.

    D. its language displays gender bias.

43. Which statement, if true, is a fact?

  A. The 2018 London New Year's Day Parade had more spectators than the 2018 NFL Super Bowl.

  B. The 2018 London New Year's Day Parade was more exciting than the 2018 NFL Super Bowl.

  C. The 2018 London New Year's Day Parade was a fantastic display of award-winning marching bands, creatively designed parade floats, and international celebrities.

  D. The 2018 London New Year's Day Parade caused greater joy and entertainment than the 2018 NFL Super Bowl.

44. Which of the following is a fact?

  A. A Mediterranean diet is easy to follow.

  B. A Mediterranean diet is the healthiest of all diets.

  C. A Mediterranean diet offers a lot of delicious foods.

  D. A Mediterranean diet is comprised of plant-based foods.

Read the following passage and answer questions 45-47.

Manny looked out the window.

"Not yet," he mumbled to himself.

He walked into the kitchen to try to distract himself. He was about to open the cookie jar when he heard a car motor.

"Now?" he ran to the window.

"Ugh," he sighed, "it is just Mr. Mendez."

Suddenly he saw it. The small, white truck he was searching for.

He burst through the door and breathlessly greeted Stanley.

Stanley smiled as he handed a stack of envelopes to Manny.

"Is this what you're looking for, son?" Stanley said with a smile.

Manny looked at the return address. *Michigan State University.*

"Yes! Thank you!" Manny cried as he bolted into his house.

"Good luck, Manny!" Stanley yelled after him.

45. From the text above, you can infer that Manny is:

  A. best friends with Stanley.

  B. anxiously awaiting the mail.

  C. very hard on himself.

  D. not a fan of Mr. Mendez.

46. Which detail does *not* provide evidence to back up the conclusion that Manny is eager for the mail to come?

A. He mumbles "not yet" to himself.

B. He is about to open the cookie jar.

C. He sighs when he sees Mr. Mendez.

D. He bursts through the door and greets Stanley.

47. Which detail from the text supports the inference that Stanley knows Manny pretty well?

A. He drives up in his truck.

B. He hands him a stack of envelopes.

C. He asks if an envelope is what he is looking for.

D. He smiles at Manny.

48. Readers make inferences when they:

A. restate the main idea of a text in different words.

B. differentiate between primary and secondary sources.

C. determine that a text is not a credible source of information.

D. use clues in the text to help them deduce implicit information.

49. Which of the following sources should be treated with skepticism even though it is primary?

A. An original work of art that has been celebrated and imitated

B. The research notes of a technician studying infectious diseases

C. An opinion article by a person who witnessed a famine firsthand

D. A 1910 article on how to treat measles by an experienced doctor

50. What type of source is the transcript of a presidential speech honoring the men and women who serve in the American Armed Forces?

A. Primary

B. Secondary

C. Tertiary

D. None of the above

51. Which term describes the most likely structure of an essay about how World War II started?

A. Technical

B. Expository

C. Cause/effect

D. Compare/contrast

52. Which of the following is an example of technical writing?

A. A user manual

B. A history book

C. An op-ed article

D. An autobiography

53. Which term describes the most likely structure of an essay proposing ways to avoid a future war?

A. Narrative

B. Persuasive

C. Description

D. Problem-solution

SECTION II. MATHEMATICS

You will have 54 minutes to complete 36 questions.

1. If a doctor is converting a medical dose for a prescription of 2 grams into milligrams (mg), what will the dosage be? (Note: 1 gram is equal to 1,000 mg).

   A. 200 mg

   B. 0.2 mg

   C. 2000 mg

   D. 20 mg

2. Change $\frac{5}{11}$ to a decimal. Simplify completely.

   A. $0.\overline{4}$

   B. $0.\overline{45}$

   C. $0.\overline{5}$

   D. $0.5\overline{4}$

3. Stacy drives an average of 60 mph for 30 minutes to get from her home to her brother's house. If her daughter takes the same route and it takes her 40 minutes to arrive, how fast on average was Stacy's daughter driving?

   A. 70 mph

   B. 40 mph

   C. 20 mph

   D. 45 mph

4. Find the area in square inches of a circular pizza with a diameter of 10.5 inches. Round to the nearest hundredth. Use 3.14 for π.

   A. 65.94

   B. 86.54

   C. 173.09

   D. 346.19

5. Convert 18 miles to kilometers. (Note: 1 mile is equal to 1.61 kilometers).

   A. 19.61 kilometers

   B. 28.98 kilometers

   C. 39.22 kilometers

   D. 57.96 kilometers

6. A service group collects trash from area roadways for four straight weeks. The amount of trash they pick up is about 19 $\frac{1}{2}$, $15\frac{1}{3}$, $20\frac{7}{10}$, and $16\frac{3}{5}$ pounds. Estimate the total number of pounds collected.

   A. 70

   B. 71

   C. 72

   D. 73

7. A parallelogram has an area of 105 square inches. Find the height in inches if the base is 15 inches in length. (Note: *A = base x height*).

   A. 3

   B. 5

   C. 7

   D. 9

8. Convert 8 liters to quarts. (Note: 1 liter is equal 1.06 quarts).

   A. 6.94 quarts

   B. 7.55 quarts

   C. 8.48 quarts

   D. 9.06 quarts

9. A cube has a side length of 10 inches. What is the surface area in square inches? (Note: The surface area of a cube is SA = 6s²).

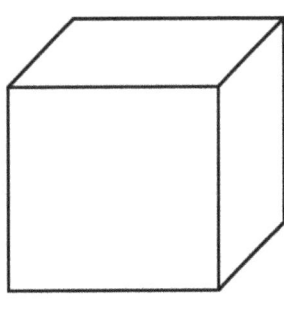

   S = 10 inches

   A. 400

   B. 600

   C. 800

   D. 1,000

10. The double line chart shows the number of points scored and points given up by a basketball team over the first 10 games. How many games did the team win?

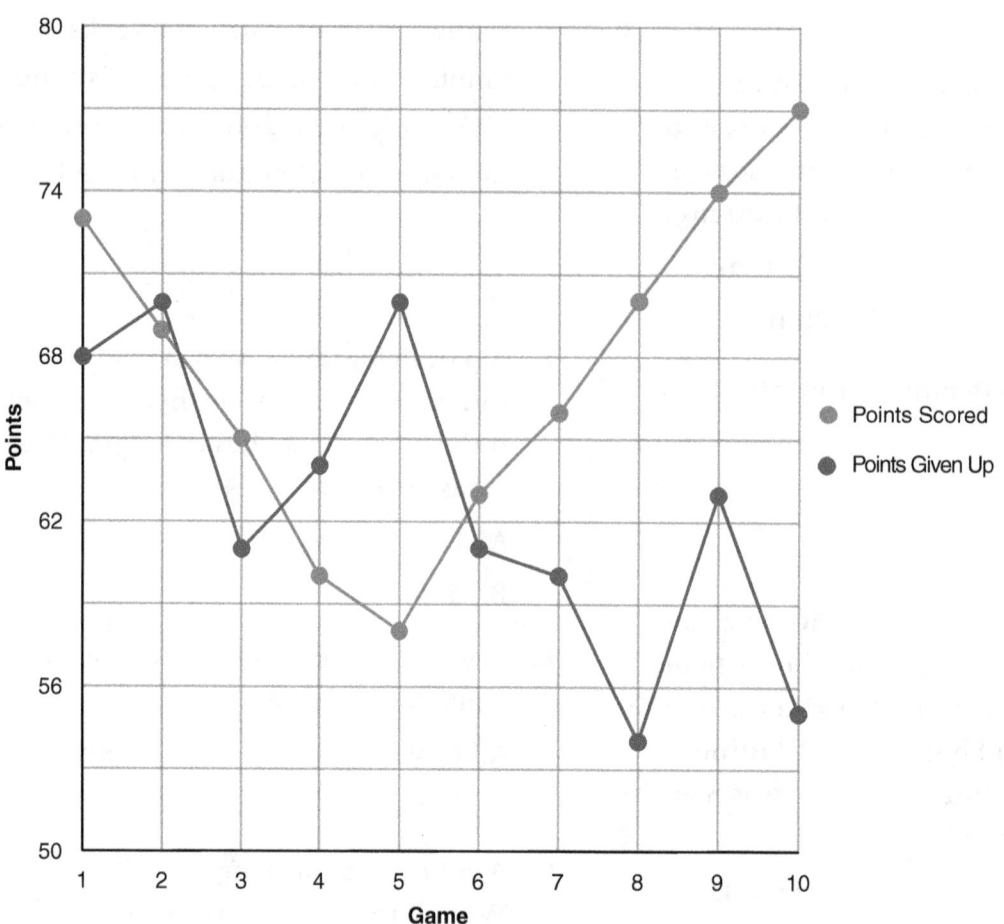

Basketball Scores

A. 5 games

B. 7 games

C. 8 games

D. 10 games

11. The founder of a new company spends part of his 40-hour work week in meetings with new investors. If he has 10 different meetings that each last 40 minutes, approximately what portion of his work time is spent in meetings?

A. $\frac{1}{10}$

B. $\frac{1}{8}$

C. $\frac{1}{6}$

D. $\frac{1}{5}$

12. Solve for the value of y when x = 4.

$y = (x^3 + 2) \div 6$

A. 3

B. 14

C. 8

D. 11

13. Multiply $2\frac{1}{4} \times 1\frac{1}{3}$.

A. 1

B. 2

C. 3

D. 4

14. The table shows the number of students in grades kindergarten through sixth grade. Select the correct bar graph for this data.

Grade	Kindergarten	1st	2nd	3rd	4th	5th	6th
Number of Students	135	150	140	155	145	165	170

A.
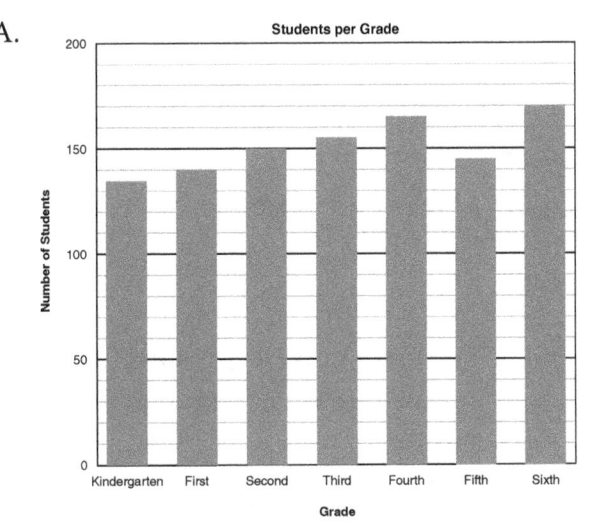

C.
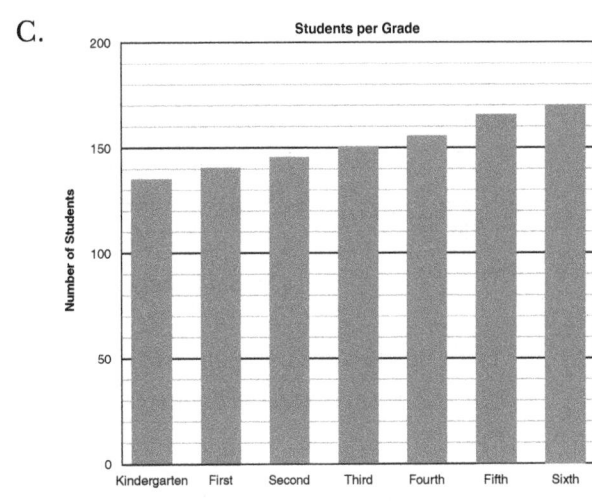

B.
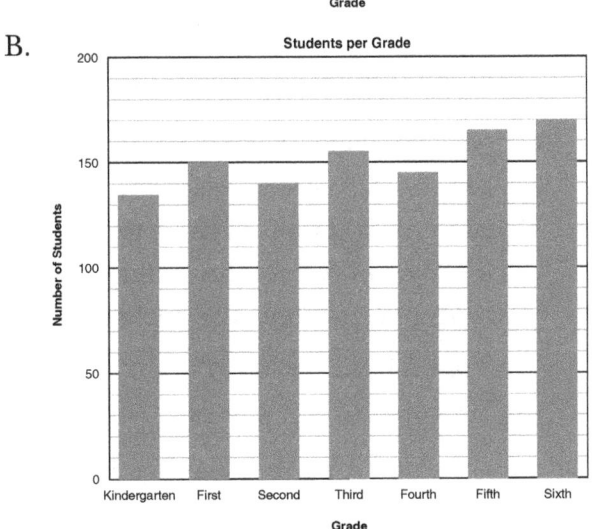

D.
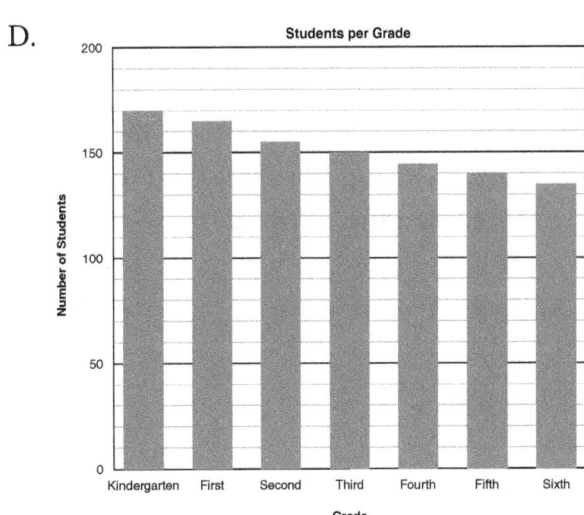

15. Alex bought a box of 500 nails to use for building a treehouse. If Alex uses $\frac{2}{5}$ of the nails for the walls and $\frac{1}{4}$ of the nails on the floor, how many nails has he used?

A. 300

C. 200

B. 475

D. 325

16. Sarah got a $\frac{21}{25}$ back on her college exam. Approximately what percentage did she earn?

A. 84%

C. 88%

B. 92%

D. 96%

17. Solve the equation for the unknown.

$3(x + 4) - 1 = 2(x + 3) - 2$

A. −7

C. 2

B. −2

D. 7

18. The box plot below shows the amount three families spent each week on groceries. Which statement describes the median and interquartile range?

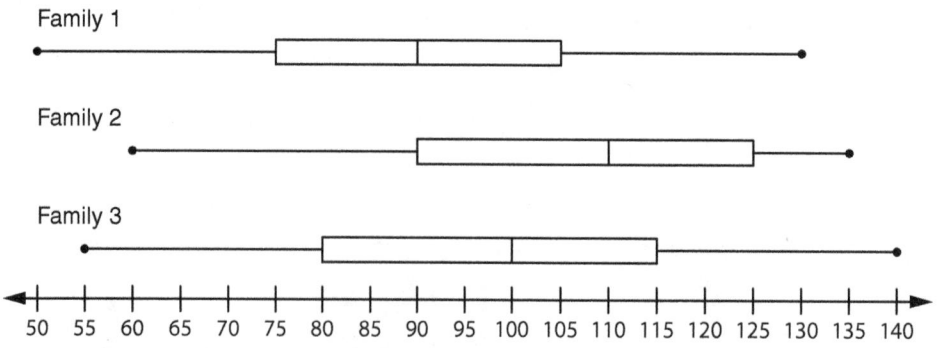

Amount Spent on Weekly Groceries

A. The median is the greatest for Family 2, but the interquartile range is greater for Family 3.

B. The median is the greatest for Family 2, but the interquartile range is the same for all families.

C. The median is the greatest for Family 1, but the interquartile range is greater for Family 3.

D. The median is the greatest for Family 1, but the interquartile range is the same for all families.

19. A student takes several 10-point math quizzes during the year. Find the mode score from the quizzes.

5, 7, 8, 6, 5, 6, 7, 8, 9, 7, 8, 10, 10, 9, 8, 7, 6, 8, 7, 9, 8, 10, 10, 9, 5, 7, 8, 9, 10, 7, 8, 9, 10

A. 7   C. 9

B. 8   D. 10

20. Solve the equation for the unknown.

$3(2x + 1)-3(x-4) = 4(2x-1)-1$

A. −4   C. 1

B. −1   D. 4

21. Celeste buys herself a fancy sports car. She put \$3,200 towards it as a down payment, and pays \$712 a month (m) for 5.5 years. Select the equation that properly represents the cost of her car.

A. $m + \$3,912 = \$50,192$

B. $\$3,912m = \$50,192$

C. $\$712m + \$3,200 = \$50,192$

D. $\$3,200m + \$712 = \$50,192$

22. A doctor leaves the hospital to go to home while driving at an average speed of 35 miles per hour. If he needs to travel 16 miles, approximately how long will it take him to arrive?

A. 30 minutes   C. 33 minutes

B. 24 minutes   D. 27 minutes

23. Which number satisfies the proportion?

$$\frac{378}{?} = \frac{18}{7}$$

   A. 18   C. 972

   B. 147   D. 2,646

24. What is the product of 8:15 and 25%?

   A. $\frac{8}{375}$ C. $\frac{15}{2}$

   B. $\frac{2}{15}$ D. $\frac{375}{8}$

25. The number 36 is what percent of 16?

   A. 31%   C. 69%

   B. 44%   D. 225%

26. A high school is using one of their training loops for a cross-country meet. The loop is equivalent to $\frac{5}{6}$ of a mile. If the participants need to run the loop 4 times, how long is the race?

   A. $2\frac{1}{2}$ C. $3\frac{1}{3}$

   B. $3\frac{5}{6}$ D. $4\frac{1}{3}$

27. Change $5\frac{3}{8}$ to a decimal. Simplify completely.

   A. 5.275   C. 5.375

   B. 5.325   D. 5.425

28. One recipe calls for $\frac{3}{4}$ cup of sugar, and another calls for $2\frac{1}{2}$ cups of sugar. The first recipe is tripled, and the second recipe is halved. How many cups of sugar are needed?

   A. 1   C. 3

   B. $1\frac{3}{4}$ D. $3\frac{1}{2}$

29. The dot plot shows the results of rolling a dice for a game. Which statement is true for the dot plot?

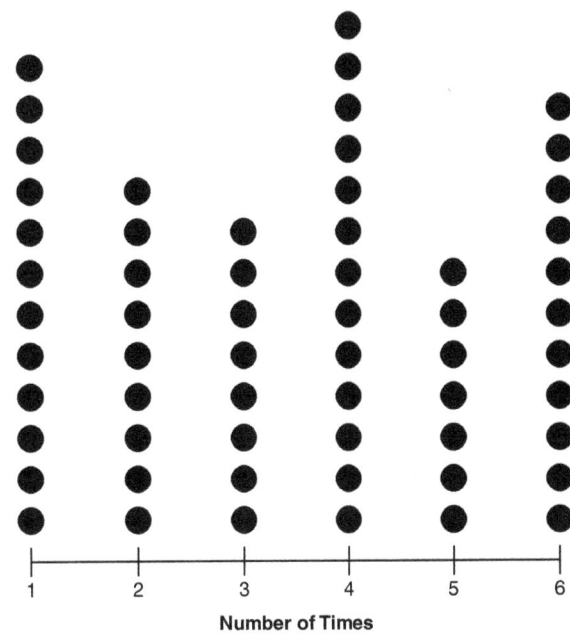

Results of Rolling a Dice

Number of Times

   A. There were 60 turns in the game.

   B. More than half of the turns were 3 or less.

   C. 1 and 6 occurred the same number of times.

   D. The difference between the lowest and highest frequency is 3.

30. Convert 750 milliliters to quarts. (Note: 1,000 milliliter is equal to 1.06 quarts.)

   A. 0.0795 quarts   C. 7.95 quarts

   B. 0.795 quarts   D. 79.5 quarts

31. Solve for x when $(9 \div 3)x = 8^2 - 1$

   A. 9   C. 7

   B. 14   D. 21

32. Find the difference.

$$1\frac{7}{9}-\frac{3}{4}$$

    A. $1\frac{1}{36}$ C. $\frac{3}{4}$

    B. $1\frac{4}{5}$ D. $\frac{11}{15}$

33. Perform the operation.

$$(5x^3 + 3x^2 - 4x + 2) + (-5x^2 - 3)$$

    A. $5x^3 - 2x^2 - 4x + 1$

    B. $5x^3 - 2x^2 - 4x - 1$

    C. $5x^3 + 2x^2 - 4x - 1$

    D. $5x^3 + 2x^2 - 4x + 1$

34. An employee is compensated two hours worth of pay for every 90 miles they travel for work. If the employee is given 18 hours of pay for travel on their paycheck, how many miles did they travel during that pay period?

    A. 324 miles   C. 900 miles

    B. 180 miles   D. 810 miles

35. A woman is determined to run an average of an 8-minute mile for her race. If she runs 12 miles in 1.75 hours, what was her average time per mile?

    A. 7:55   C. 7:45

    B. 8:30   D. 8:45

36. Divide.

$$2\frac{7}{9} \div 2\frac{1}{3}$$

    A. $1\frac{1}{9}$ C. $1\frac{7}{27}$

    B. $1\frac{4}{21}$ D. $1\frac{7}{9}$

SECTION III. SCIENCE

You have 63 minutes to complete 53 questions.

1. Which of the following is a function of epithelial tissue?

   A. Secreting toxins

   B. Expelling mucus

   C. Acting as barriers

   D. Secreting hormones

2. The lips are _____ to the neck.

   A. anterior   C. inferior

   B. deep   D. superior

3. The shoulder is _____ to the fingertips.

   A. distal   C. proximal

   B. inferior   D. superficial

4. Which happens as a result of a diastole?

   A. The left ventricle flows blood to the aorta.

   B. Oxygenated blood drains into the left ventricle.

   C. Blood travels from the arteries to the arterioles.

   D. The pulmonary artery flows blood to the left atrium.

5. Which blood group indicates the absence of the Rh factor?

   A. AB   C. B+

   B. A-   D. O

6. Which of the following is an effect of aging on hormone secretion?

   A. Weak teeth

   B. Loss of appetite

   C. Trouble sleeping

   D. Loss of body hair

7. In stressful situations, acetylcholine is produced. Which intercellular chemical signal is responsible for this action?

   A. Autocrine

   B. Neuromodulator

   C. Paracrine

   D. Pheromone

8. The pancreas is technically an organ of the exocrine system. How does it benefit the digestive system?

   A. It secretes mucus.

   B. It secretes glycogen.

   C. It secretes hydrochloric acid.

   D. It secretes digestive enzymes.

9. Which of the following is the correct path of food through the digestive system?

   A. Oral cavity → pharynx → esophagus → stomach → small intestine → large intestine

   B. Oral cavity → pharynx → esophagus → stomach → liver → small intestine → large intestine

   C. Oral cavity → pharynx → esophagus → stomach → liver → pancreas → small intestine → large intestine

   D. Oral cavity → pharynx → esophagus → stomach → liver → gallbladder → pancreas → small intestine → large intestine

10. In what order does food pass through the parts of the small intestine?

    A. Duodenum → jejunum → ileum

    B. Duodenum → ileum → jejunum

    C. Ileum → jejunum → duodenum

    D. Jejunum → duodenum → ileum

11. Squamous cell carcinoma affects cells in the stratum _____.

    A. basale   C. lucidum

    B. granulosum   D. spinosum

12. If a person wants to slow down the development of wrinkly skin, which of the following activities could be performed?

    A. Improve mitotic epidermal cell division

    B. Receive fat injections in the hypodermis

    C. Add collagen to the stratum corneum layer

    D. Slow down keratin production in the dermis

13. Platelets are important because they

    A. give blood its natural color.

    B. repair broken blood vessels.

    C. transport nutrients to the cells.

    D. protect the body against infection.

14. Why is a vaccinated person said to be immunized against a particular disease?

    A. The number of helper T cells has increased.

    B. The number of macrophages has increased.

    C. Antibodies used to fight that disease have been produced.

    D. Histamines used to fight that disease have been produced.

15. What structure is reenergized with ATP?

    A. Actin

    B. Myosin

    C. Myofibril

    D. Sarcomere

16. What happens after myosin heads attach to thin actin myofilaments?

    A. Crossbridges are formed.

    B. Molecules of ATP are released.

    C. The myosin head is reenergized.

    D. Calcium ion concentration increases.

17. Which is a characteristic of the epimysium?

    A. Groups muscle fibers at joint sites

    B. Protects muscles as they rub against bones

    C. Is the deepest layer of connective tissue in skeletal muscle

    D. Contains capillaries and nerves to facilitate contraction

18. Which structure provides bones the largest freedom of movement?

    A. Tendon   C. Synovial joint

    B. Ligament   D. Smooth muscle

19. Where does an axon bind to release hormones in the body?

    A. gland
    B. dendrite
    C. cell body
    D. muscle cell

20. Neuroglia are different from neurons because they

    A. participate in synaptic transmission.
    B. maintain sustained action potentials.
    C. transmit electric signals as messages.
    D. provide a form of protection and support.

21. When do vesicles contract and move to the presynaptic membrane?

    A. After calcium ions flood the axon bulb
    B. Exactly as an axon connects to a dendrite
    C. Before voltage gated sodium channels open
    D. While an electric signal travels down an axon

22. Menopause occurs _____.

    A. earlier in males than in females
    B. in females at an average age of 51
    C. just after the end of embryogenesis
    D. during the second week of each menstrual cycle

23. During childbirth, muscular action in the _____ is primarily responsible for pushing the baby out of the mother's body.

    A. cervix
    B. uterus
    C. vagina
    D. vulva

24. Which body system plays a direct role in supplying oxygen to cells and eliminating carbon dioxide from cells?

    A. Cardiovascular
    B. Nervous
    C. Respiratory
    D. Urinary

25. What process begins with red blood cells giving up oxygen to other cells in the body?

    A. Air conduction
    B. Cellular respiration
    C. Internal respiration
    D. Pulmonary ventilation

26. What structure changes shape during the mechanics of breathing?

    A. Bronchiole
    B. Diaphragm
    C. Nose
    D. Pharynx

27. What is a characteristic of compact bone?

    A. Site of hematopoiesis
    B. Made of dense connective tissue
    C. Contains the osteocyte bone cells
    D. Consists of several openings or pores

28. Where are osteons found?

    A. Next to an osteocyte
    B. Inside compact bone
    C. Above the periosteum
    D. On the surface of spongy bone

29. Which of the following consists primarily of fat cells?

    A. Epiphysis

    B. Periosteum

    C. Yellow marrow

    D. Articular cartilage

30. After urine flows through one sphincter at the start of the bladder, this fluid flows through the

    A. urethra naturally because of gravity.

    B. urethra after two sphincters contract.

    C. second sphincter under voluntary control.

    D. collecting ducts at the base of the renal tubule.

31. What does the skeletal system provide?

    A. Circulation

    B. Energy

    C. Immunity

    D. Support

32. Which of the following is permeable to water when the ADH is present?

    A. loop of Henle

    B. collecting duct

    C. renal corpuscle

    D. proximal convoluted tubule

33. Which metabolic pathway generates the most ATP?

    A. Glycolysis

    B. Citric acid cycle

    C. Gluconeogenesis

    D. Oxidative phosphorylation

34. What is a control variable?

    A. The variable that is used for comparisons

    B. The responding variable in an experiment

    C. The manipulated variable in an experiment

    D. The variable that is measured or able to be changed

35. What is a monomer of a carbohydrate?

    A. Oil

    B. RNA

    C. Glycerol

    D. Monosaccharide

36. Which process is anabolic?

    A. Glycolysis

    B. Lipid synthesis

    C. Protein degradation

    D. Oxidative phosphorylation

37. What is the basis for classifying an organism as either an autotroph or a heterotroph?

    A. The way an organism obtains its energy

    B. The organism's ranking in the taxonomic system

    C. The type of ecosystem in which an organism lives

    D. Whether the organism is unicellular or multicellular

38. Which organisms are heterotrophs?

    A. Algae   C. Bacteria

    B. Bears   D. Flowers

39. Which organism most likely produces offspring asexually?

    A. Bacteria   C. Humans

    B. Birds   D. Lions

40. DNA _____ during the synthesis phase in mitosis.

    A. splits in half

    B. triples in size

    C. doubles in size

    D. breaks into small pieces

41. Sister chromatids and centromeres are found in a _____ chromosome.

    A. replicated

    B. duplicated

    C. histone absent

    D. loosely condensed

42. Right before cell division, a DNA molecule and its associated proteins

    A. coil tightly.

    B. stretch out.

    C. form a double helix.

    D. wrap around each other.

43. Transcription manufactures _____.

    A. proteins

    B. enzymes

    C. ribonucleic acid

    D. deoxyribonucleic acid

44. According to Mendel's observations, which of the following is a theory of heredity?

    A. Individuals receive one allele from each parent.

    B. Genotype determines the physical appearance of a person.

    C. Parents transmit genetic traits directly to offspring without genes.

    D. All phenotypic traits come from either the mom or dad, but not both.

45. What is DNA packaged in?

    A. Chromosomes

    B. Nucleotides

    C. Centromeres

    D. Phosphate

46. During which of the following phase changes will a substance absorb energy?

    A. Condensation

    B. Deposition

    C. Freezing

    D. Sublimation

47. Which analysis describes the results shown in the following image?

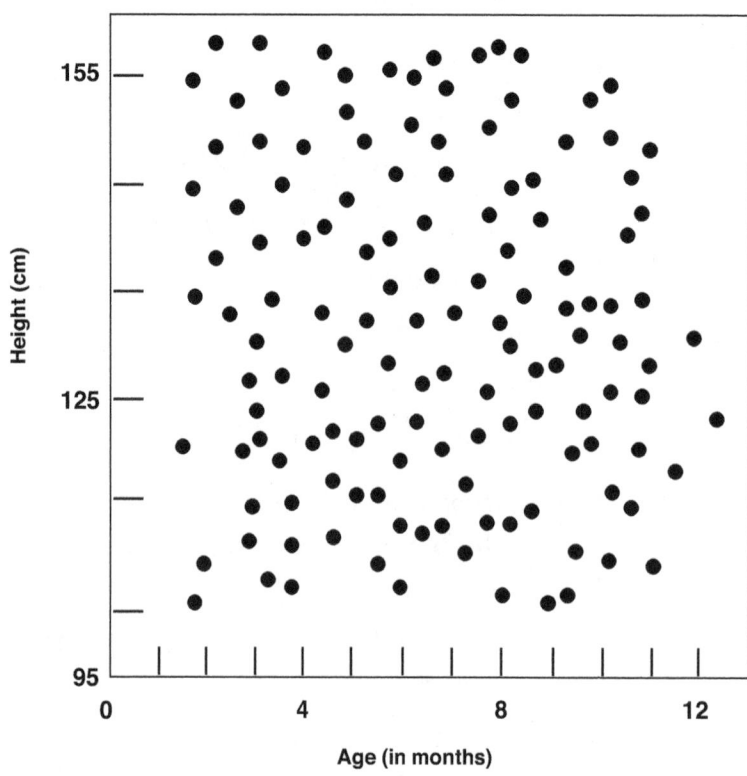

Relationship Between A Boy's Height and Age
(simulated data)

Height (cm)

Age (in months)

A. As a baby gets older, he gets taller.

B. Birth month is independent of height.

C. Older boys are taller than younger boys

D. A baby's height stays the same every month.

48. An atom has 3 protons, 4 neutrons, and 3 electrons. Which element is it?

A. Beryllium C. Lithium

B. Carbon D. Neon

49. Zinc-64 is one possible isotope of the element zinc. Which of the atoms described below is a different isotope of zinc?

A. 34 protons, 34 neutrons, 34 electrons

B. 34 protons, 30 neutrons, 34 electrons

C. 30 protons, 36 neutrons, 30 electrons

D. 64 protons, 34 neutrons, 34 electrons

50. Which of the following elements is in the same family as calcium?

A. Potassium C. Strontium

B. Scandium D. Yttrium

51. Which of the following pairs of elements contains two elements in the same group?

A. Iron and cobalt

B. Fluorine and bromine

C. Hydrogen and helium

D. Sodium and magnesium

52. The melting point of a substance is an example of a(n) _____ property.

   A. chemical   C. intensive

   B. extensive   D. reactive

53. Which of the following is being described?

   The molecules move around more, and the particles are unable to hold together as tightly. They break apart, and the solid becomes a liquid.

   A. Deposition   C. Melting

   B. Freezing   D. Sublimation

SECTION IV. ENGLISH AND LANGUAGE USAGE

You have 28 minutes to complete 28 questions.

1. **Which of the following sentences is correct?**

   A. They used to live in the pacific northwest.

   B. They used to live in the Pacific northwest.

   C. They used to live in the pacific Northwest.

   D. They used to live in the Pacific Northwest.

2. **Which of the following sentences is correct?**

   A. No; I did not do that.

   B. Yes: I ate the leftovers.

   C. No, I am not leaving yet.

   D. Yes I finished my homework.

3. **What is the correct plural of waltz?**

   A. Waltzs   C. Waltzies

   B. Waltzes   D. Waltzzes

4. **Which of the following nouns correctly completes this sentence?**

   We can use these _____ to cut these fillets of _____.

   A. knives, salmon

   B. knifes, salmon

   C. knifes, salmons

   D. knives, salmons

5. **What is the role of the pronoun *him* in a sentence?**

   A. Object   C. Possessive

   B. Subject   D. Any of these

6. **Which word in the following sentence is an adjective?**

   Washington, Jefferson, and Adams were founding fathers of the United States.

   A. and   C. fathers

   B. founding   D. of

7. **How many prepositions are in the following sentence?**

   The athletes traveled from Boston to Dallas for the competition.

   A. 0   C. 2

   B. 1   D. 3

8. **Which of the following verbs correctly completes this sentence?**

   Katharina didn't ____ her job as an accountant, so she decided to change careers.

   A. like   C. liken

   B. likes   D. liked

9. **Which subject is third person singular?**

   A. I   C. We

   B. He   D. You

10. **Which of the following verbs correctly completes this sentence?**

    Neither Grandma nor Aunt Lucy ____ where the old photos are.

    A. know   C. known

    B. knows   D. knowing

11. Which of the following subjects correctly agrees with the verb "honor" in this sentence?

On Memorial Day, which is the last Monday in May, Americans <u>honor</u> those who have died for their country.

A. Memorial Day   C. Americans

B. which   D. died

12. Fill in the blank with the correct coordinating conjunction.

Julia wanted the new iPhone, _____ she could not afford it.

A. so   C. but

B. or   D. and

13. Identify the type of clause.

The reporter stumbled over his words.

A. Coordinate clause

B. Dependent clause

C. Subordinate clause

D. Independent clause

14. Which of the following options correctly fixes the fragment below?

Rather than go skiing.

A. Rather than go skiing Sasha opted to go snowboarding.

B. Rather than go skiing, Sasha opted to go snowboarding.

C. Rather than go skiing. Sasha opted to go snowboarding.

D. Rather than go skiing, so Sasha opted to go snowboarding.

15. Which of the following options would complete the above sentence to make it a simple sentence?

Eating salmon once a week

_____.

A. is a healthy choice

B. is good, and it is healthy

C. is healthy it is a good choice

D. is healthy while still being good

16. Which of the following options would give the sentence below a parallel structure?

Traveling gives people memorable experiences, exposes them to different cultures, and _____.

A. broadens their perspective

B. to broaden their perspective

C. broadening their perspective

D. will broaden their perspective

17. In which of the following situations would it be best to use informal language?

A. Buying a suit

B. A birthday party

C. A meeting at work

D. Going to a work lunch

18. Which of the following sentences uses the MOST formal language?

A. This essay claims that sugar is bad for people.

B. I think that sugar is bad for people.

C. I believe that sugar is bad for people.

D. I say that sugar is bad for people.

19. Which of the following context clues correctly helps you define the word "stall" in this sentence?

Suddenly braking too quickly can stall a car's engine, causing it to stop working altogether.

A. "suddenly braking"

B. "too quickly"

C. "stop working"

D. "altogether"

20. Which of the following context clues correctly helps you define the word "apathetic" in this sentence?

The students seemed apathetic about the vandalism since they walked nonchalantly by the graffiti-covered wall.

A. "vandalism"

B. "walking"

C. "nonchalantly "

D. "graffiti-covered"

21. Which of the following words in this sentence has more than one meaning?

Rice is a dietary staple in a lot of Asian countries.

A. Dietary   C. Asian

B. Staple   D. Countries

22. Which of the following is the meaning of "produce" as used in this sentence?

The auto company plans to produce a luxury line of electric cars.

A. Cause to happen

B. Manufacture or build

C. Show or provide for consideration

D. Administer the financial aspects of a movie

23. Which of the following is the meaning of "advocate" as used in this sentence?

Martha is a passionate advocate for civil rights and spends all her time fighting for the cause.

A. Expert   C. Admirer

B. Teacher   D. Supporter

24. *Natal* means relating to

A. life.   C. birth.

B. age.   D. health.

25. Which of the following root words means "sound"?

A. ped   C. phon

B. vis   D. post

26. Which of the following prefixes means "after"?

A. peri-   C. ante-

B. com-   D. post-

27. **Which of the following is the meaning of "polytheistic" as used in this sentence?**

His religion is characterized as polytheistic, which is unlike most other religions.

A. Believing in many gods

B. Practicing infrequently

C. Consisting of only men

D. Having its own language

28. **What is the best definition of the word** *spherical?*

A. Hard   C. Rough

B. Round   D. Absorbent

TEAS Practice Exam 5
Answer Key with Explanatory Answers

Section I. Reading

1. B. The topic of this paragraph is dress codes. Enforcing a specific school uniform is related to this topic, but is not covered in detail in this passage. **Skill: Main Ideas, Topic Sentences, and Supporting Details.**

2. A. The first sentence of this paragraph leads the reader toward the main idea, which is expressed next in a topic sentence about the benefits of school dress codes. **Skill: Main Ideas, Topic Sentences, and Supporting Details.**

3. C. A description of a student wearing clothing that does not meet dress code requirements would function as a supporting detail in this paragraph about the school dress codes. **Skill: Main Ideas, Topic Sentences, and Supporting Details.**

4. B. A flowchart is a graphic used to show a sequence of actions or decisions involved in a complex process. **Skill: Summarizing Text and Using Text Features.**

5. C. A bar graph uses rectangles to convey differences between numerical values at a glance. **Skill: Summarizing Text and Using Text Features.**

6. D. Body paragraphs come in the middle of an essay, after the topic is introduced. They must relate clearly to the main point and avoid veering off in unexpected directions. **Skill: The Writing Process.**

7. C. An introductory paragraph gives readers everything they need to know to follow the ideas in the rest of an essay. **Skill: The Writing Process.**

8. D. Texts that say why one thing is better than another—including advertising texts—usually use a compare/contrast structure. **Skill: The Writing Process.**

9. A. An outline organizes ideas into the rough order they'll follow in a piece of writing. **Skill: The Writing Process.**

10. D. The word *fragrance* has a positive connotation and would help show the author's positive attitude toward the woman and her perfume. **Skill: Essay Revision and Transitions.**

11. B. The word *stench* has a negative connotation and would help show the author's negative attitude toward the woman and her perfume. **Skill: Essay Revision and Transitions.**

12. C. Revising for inclusivity means eliminating stereotypically gendered language use. Here, the original author uses "man" to refer to all of humankind. **Skill: Essay Revision and Transitions.**

3. A. The word *get* is both informal and imprecise and could be replaced, in this context, with *understand*. The phrase *took out* can similarly be replaced with the more formal *removed*. **Skill: Essay Revision and Transitions.**

4. B. There are times when it is best to avoid gendered pronouns, but there is no need to avoid them all the time. And rhetorically effective writing is not directly connected to gendered language. **Skill: Essay Revision and Transitions.**

5. D. The sentences above would be best served with an example transition and an addition transition. **Skill: Tone, Mood, and Transition Words.**

6. C. The transition is the word that links the two ideas: *thus*. This word shows how the two sentences have a cause-and-effect relationship. **Skill: Tone, Mood, and Transition Words.**

7. C. The transition is the word that links the two ideas: *also*. The word *however* here is not a transition word indicating contrast; it's an adverb meaning "in whichever way." **Skill: Tone, Mood, and Transition Words.**

8. A. Setting details and details that suggest theme are some of the most important tools or establishing mood. **Skill: Tone, Mood, and Transition Words.**

9. A. Tone is the author's attitude, and mood is the reader's reaction. Both terms would be necessary to discuss any differences between the two. **Skill: Tone, Mood, and Transition Words.**

20. A. A transition helps link ideas within a text. Common transitions include words and phrases like "first," "furthermore," and "for example." **Skill: Tone, Mood, and Transition Words.**

21. C. Transitions are not meant to tell the reader the mood of a text (and since mood is the reader's emotional reaction, it's not something that can be dictated to the reader anyway). **Skill: Tone, Mood, and Transition Words.**

22. D. A transition between these two sentences would likely suggest contrast. Good choices would be words like *nevertheless* or *however*. **Skill: Tone, Mood, and Transition Words.**

23. A. Passage 1 is intended to inform readers about electroconvulsive therapy. **Skill: Understanding the Author's Purpose, Point of View, and Rhetorical Strategies.**

24. C. The second paragraph of Passage 1 makes opinion statements about what doctors should do. This is a sign of persuasive writing. **Skill: Understanding the Author's Purpose, Point of View, and Rhetorical Strategies.**

25. D. Passage 2 tells a story, which is meant to entertain. **Skill: Understanding the Author's Purpose, Point of View, and Rhetorical Strategies.**

26. D. Passage 1 says that electroconvulsive therapy is "a genuine option for patients whose symptoms do not improve with medication." This suggests that medication should be tried first. **Skill: Understanding the Author's Purpose, Point of View, and Rhetorical Strategies.**

27. C. The detail about electroconvulsive therapy as "a genuine option for patients whose symptoms do not improve with medication" suggests that patients should try an option like medication first, before contemplating electroconvulsive therapy. **Skill: Understanding the Author's Purpose, Point of View, and Rhetorical Strategies.**

28. A. The author of Passage 2 is aware that many people have negative preconceived ideas about electroconvulsive therapy. This is true of the author of Passage 2, who does not inform herself about the facts of the situation. **Skill: Understanding the Author's Purpose, Point of View, and Rhetorical Strategies.**

29. D. The author of Passage 1 specifically recommends extra care in communication about electroconvulsive therapy. The doctor in Passage 2 does not seem to make any extra effort to differentiate between myth and reality. **Skill: Understanding the Author's Purpose, Point of View, and Rhetorical Strategies.**

30. A. The author of Passage 2 describes doctors blocking her "direct path to the door," which suggests that she feels trapped in the room. This suggests a negative, fearful outlook which is further reinforced by the comment about Big Doctor being "sadistic." **Skill: Understanding the Author's Purpose, Point of View, and Rhetorical Strategies.**

31. B. The author of Passage 1 uses primarily facts and logic, although she could strengthen her points by clearly identifying sources or establishing her credentials. **Skill: Understanding the Author's Purpose, Point of View, and Rhetorical Strategies.**

32. C. An index lists the subtopics of a book along with page numbers where those topics will be covered. **Skill: Evaluating and Integrating Data.**

33. D. The table of contents gives a broad picture of what a text covers in each chapter, so it is a good first place to look when you're determining whether or not a book is useful for research. Scanning subheadings and consulting the index may also be useful. **Skill: Evaluating and Integrating Data.**

34. C. Horizontal lines on a chart are called rows, and vertical lines are called legends. Using this terminology, it is possible to describe the spaces on the chart (e.g., "What is the value in the fourth column of the second row?"). **Skill: Evaluating and Integrating Data.**

35. D. Many maps are equipped with a key or legend to show what their symbols and markings mean. **Skill: Evaluating and Integrating Data.**

36. B. The argument that prison nursery programs can be beneficial is an opinion statement because it makes a judgment. **Skill: Facts, Opinions, and Evaluating an Argument.**

37. **B.** The statement makes a factual statement about how people said they felt. This makes it a fact even though it contains opinion information. **Skill: Facts, Opinions, and Evaluating an Argument.**

38. **C.** The main argument in this passage is that it may be beneficial to both mothers and babies if women who give birth in prison are allowed to keep their children with them. One assumption behind the passage is that society must promote the health and safety of children, but this is not the main argument. **Skill: Facts, Opinions, and Evaluating an Argument.**

39. **D.** The passage states explicitly that the idea of raising children in prison is controversial, so this is not an assumption. It does assume that our society should attempt to help children born to mothers in prison. **Skill: Facts, Opinions, and Evaluating an Argument.**

40. **B.** The sentence about putting babies in jail uses its own reason to defend its argument. It needs to provide evidence instead. **Skill: Facts, Opinions, and Evaluating an Argument.**

41. **A.** The paragraph about benefits to mothers shows that mothers who participate in the prison nursery program have better outcomes. It suggests but does not prove that their participation in the program is the cause of these outcomes. **Skill: Facts, Opinions, and Evaluating an Argument.**

42. **B.** The sentences use a form of faulty reasoning called either/or reasoning. They suggest that there are only two possible ways for society to respond to the issue of babies being born in prison when in fact there are many. **Skill: Facts, Opinions, and Evaluating an Argument.**

43. **A.** All of these statements contain beliefs or feelings that are subject to interpretation except the statement about the number of people attending the 2018 London New Year's Day Parade compared to the 2018 NFL Super Bowl. This is a verifiable piece of information, or a fact. **Skill: Facts, Opinions, and Evaluating an Argument.**

44. **D.** The statement that is a fact is that a Mediterranean diet is comprised of plant-based foods. This is not an opinion but a piece of information that is verifiably true. **Skill: Facts, Opinions, and Evaluating an Argument.**

45. **B.** Manny is anxiously awaiting the mail. You know this because he "looked out the window," says, "not yet," and bursts "through the door" after he sees the "small, white truck." **Skill: Understanding Primary Sources, Making Inferences, and Drawing Conclusions.**

46. **B.** Manny opening the cookie jar does not explicitly show that he is eager for the mail to come. **Skill: Understanding Primary Sources, Making Inferences, and Drawing Conclusions.**

47. C. When Stanley shows Manny the envelope from Michigan State and says with a smile, "Is this what you're looking for, son?" it shows that he knows Manny is eagerly waiting to hear from colleges. This proves that he knows Manny pretty well since he knows what's going on in his life. **Skill: Understanding Primary Sources, Making Inferences, and Drawing Conclusions.**

48. D. Readers make inferences when they deduce implicit information in a text. **Skill: Understanding Primary Sources, Making Inferences, and Drawing Conclusions.**

49. D. A 1910 article on medicine is highly outdated. Even if the writer is an experienced doctor, the advice presented would likely not be worth following. **Skill: Understanding Primary Sources, Making Inferences, and Drawing Conclusions.**

50. A. A transcript of a speech is a primary source. **Skill: Understanding Primary Sources, Making Inferences, and Drawing Conclusions.**

51. C. The structure of a text is its organizational scheme, not its category. Of the options above, a cause/effect structure is most likely. **Skill: Types of Passages, Text Structures, Genre and Theme.**

52. A. A user manual describes a complex mechanism and the processes for maintaining it, so it is a technical text. **Skill: Types of Passages, Text Structures, Genre and Theme.**

53. D. The structure of a text is its organizational scheme, not its category. Of the options, a problem-solution structure is most likely. **Skill: Types of Passages, Text Structures, Genre and Theme.**

Section II. Mathematics

1. C. One gram is equal to 1,000 milligrams, so 2 grams is equivalent to 2,000 milligrams. **Skill: Solving Real World Mathematical Problems.**

2. B. The correct answer is $0.\overline{45}$ because $\frac{5}{11} = 5.00 \div 11 = 0.\overline{45}$. **Skill: Decimals and Fractions.**

3. D. Since Stacy was driving 60mph and she arrived home in 30 minutes, 60 mph × ½hour = 30 miles. Therefore, Stacy's daughter drove 30 miles as well. Since her daughter was driving at a rate of 45mph, 30 miles divided by 40 minutes would yield and average speed of 45mph. **Skill: Ratios, Proportions, and Percentages.**

4. B. The correct solution is 86.54. The radius is 5.25 centimeters and $A = \pi r^2 \approx 3.14(5.25)^2 \approx 3.14(27.5625) \approx 86.54$ square inches. **Skill: Circles.**

5. B. The correct solution is 28.98 kilometers. $18\ mi \times \frac{1.61\ km}{1\ mi} = 28.98\ km$. **Skill: Standards of Measure.**

6. D. The correct solution is 73. The estimated weights are 20, 15, 21, and 17 pounds, and the total weight is about 73 pounds. **Skill: Solving Real World Mathematical Problems.**

7. C. The correct solution is 7. Substitute the values into the formula, $105 = 15h$ and divide both sides of the equation by 15, $h = 7$ inches. **Skill: Similarity, Right Triangles, and Trigonometry.**

8. C. The correct solution is 8.48 quarts. $8\,L \times \frac{1.06\,qt}{1\,L} = 8.48\,qt$. **Skill: Standards of Measure.**

9. B. The correct solution is 600. Substitute the values into the formula and simplify using the order of operations, $SA = 6s^2 = 6(10^2) = 6(100) = 600$ square inches. **Skill: Similarity, Right Triangles, and Trigonometry.**

10. B. The correct solution is the team won 7 games because the team scored more points than the opponents in these games. **Skill: Interpreting Graphics.**

11. C. The founder spends a total of 400 minutes of his work week in meetings because 10 meetings x 40 minutes = 400 minutes. There are a total of 2400 minutes in a 40-hour work week and $\frac{400}{2400} = \frac{1}{6}$. **Skill: Multiplication and Division of Fractions.**

12. D. The correct solution is 11 because $x^3 = 64 + 2 = 66 \div 6 = 11$. **Skill: Equations with One Variable.**

13. C. The correct solution is 3 because $\frac{9}{4} \times \frac{4}{3} = \frac{36}{12} = 3$. **Skill: Multiplication and Division of Fractions.**

14. B. The correct solution is B because the number of students for each grade is correct. **Skill: Interpreting Graphics.**

15. D. Alex used 325 nails because converting the fractions shows that he used $\frac{8}{20} + \frac{5}{20} = \frac{13}{20}$ of the nails. $\frac{500}{1} \times \frac{13}{20} = 325$ nails. **Skill: Multiplication and Division of Fractions.**

16. A. Sarah earned an 84% on her exam because $\frac{21}{25} = \frac{84}{100}$ or 84%. **Skill: Ratios, Proportions, and Percentages.**

17. A. The correct solution is −7.

$3x + 12 - 1 = 2x + 6 - 2$	Apply the distributive property.
$3x + 11 = 2x + 4$	Combine like terms on both sides of the equation.
$x + 11 = 4$	Subtract $2x$ from both sides of the equation.
$x = -7$	Subtract 11 from both sides of the equation.

Skill: Equations with One Variable.

18. D. The correct solution is the median is the greatest for Family 2, but the interquartile range is the same for all families. The median is $110 for Family 2, but the interquartile range is $35 for each family. **Skill: Interpreting Categorical and Quantitative Data.**

19. B. The correct solution is 8. The quiz score of 8 occurred 8 times, which is the mode. **Skill: Interpreting Graphics.**

20. D. The correct solution is 4.

$6x + 3-3x + 12 = 8x-4-1$ Apply the distributive property.

$3x + 15 = 8x-5$ Combine like terms on both sides of the equation.

$-5x + 15 = -5$ Subtract $8x$ from both sides of the equation.

$-5x = -20$ Subtract 15 from both sides of the equation

$x = 4$ Divide both sides of the equation by -5.

Skill: Equations with One Variable.

21. C. Celeste's sports car costs $50,192 because 5.5 years of payments = 66 x $712 per month = $46,992 + $3,200 down payment = $50,192 total. The equation that properly represents this cost is $712m + \$3,200 = \$50,192$. **Skill: Solving Real World Mathematical Problems.**

22. D. It will take the doctor 27 minutes to get home because $\frac{35\ miles}{60\ minutes} = \frac{16\ miles}{27\ minutes}$. **Skill: Solving Real World Mathematical Problems.**

23. B. The number 147 satisfies the proportion. First, divide 378 by 18 to get 21. Then, multiply 21 by 7 to get 147. Check your answer by dividing 147 by 7: the quotient is also 21, so 147 satisfies the proportion. **Skill: Ratios, Proportions, and Percentages.**

24. B. Ratios act just like fractions, so this product is the product of $\frac{8}{15}$ and 25% (which is equal to $\frac{1}{4}$). The answer is $\frac{8}{60} = \frac{2}{15}$. **Skill: Ratios, Proportions, and Percentages.**

25. D. The fraction $\frac{36}{16}$ is 225%, meaning 36 is 225% of 16. **Skill: Ratios, Proportions, and Percentages.**

26. C. The participants run a total of $3\frac{1}{3}$ miles because $\frac{5}{6}$ x $\frac{4}{1} = \frac{20}{6} = 3\frac{1}{3}$ miles. **Skill: Multiplication and Division of Fractions.**

27. C. The correct answer is 5.375 because $\frac{3}{8} = 3.000 \div 8 = 0.375$. **Skill: Decimals and Fractions.**

28. D. The correct solution is $3\frac{1}{2}$ because $\frac{3}{4}(3) + 2\frac{1}{2}(\frac{1}{2}) = \frac{3}{4}(\frac{3}{1}) + \frac{5}{2}(\frac{1}{2}) = \frac{9}{4} + \frac{5}{4} = \frac{14}{4} = \frac{7}{2} = 3\frac{1}{2}$ cups of sugar. **Skill: Solving Real World Mathematical Problems.**

29. A. The correct solution is there were 60 turns in the game. The sum of the results is 12 + 9 + 8 + 13 + 7 + 11, which is 60 turns. **Skill: Interpreting Categorical and Quantitative Data.**

30. B. The correct solution is 0.795 quarts. $750\ mL \times \frac{1\ L}{1,000\ mL} \times \frac{1.06\ qt}{1\ L} = \frac{795}{1000} = 0.795\ qt$. **Skill: Standards of Measure.**

31. D. The correct solution is 21 because the equation simplifies to 3x = 64 − 1 = 3x = 63 and x = 21. **Skill: Equations with One Variable.**

32. A. The correct solution is $1\frac{1}{36}$ because $1\frac{7}{9}-\frac{3}{4} = \frac{16}{9}-\frac{3}{4} = \frac{64}{36} - \frac{27}{36} = \frac{37}{36} = 1\frac{1}{36}$. **Skill: Addition and Subtraction of Fractions.**

33. B. The correct solution is $5x^3-2x^2-4x-1$.

$(5x^3 + 3x^2-4x + 2) + (-5x^2-3) = 5x^3 + (3x^2-5x^2)-4x + (2-3)$

$$= 5x^3 - 2x^2 - 4x - 1$$

Skill: Polynomials.

34. D. The employee traveled 810 miles because $\frac{90\ miles}{2\ hours} = \frac{X}{18\ hours}$ and x = 810 miles. Skill: Ratios, Proportions, and Percentages.

35. D. There are 60 minutes in an hour, so 1.75 hours converts to 1 hour and 45 minutes or a total of 105 minutes. Dividing her total time by the number of miles she ran, it took 8.75 or $8\frac{3}{4}$ minutes per mile. This number can be converted to 8 minutes and 45 seconds per mile. Skill: Decimals and Fractions.

36. B. The correct answer is $1\frac{4}{21}$ because $\frac{25}{9} \div \frac{7}{3} = \frac{25}{9} \times \frac{3}{7} = \frac{75}{63} = 1\frac{12}{63} = 1\frac{4}{21}$. Skill: Multiplication and Division of Fractions.

Section III. Science

1. C. Functions of the epithelial tissue include protecting underlying structures, acting as barriers, permitting the passage of substances, and secreting substances, but not toxins or hormones. Skill: Organization of the Human Body.

2. D. *Superior* means a structure is above another. The lips are above the neck. Skill: Organization of the Human Body.

3. C. The term *proximal* means something is closer to the point of attachment to the body than another structure. The shoulder is closer to the torso than the fingertips are. Skill: Organization of the Human Body.

4. B. A diastole occurs when there is a period of relaxation and the chambers fill with blood. For oxygenated blood to drain into the left ventricle, the left atrium must relax and fill with blood. Skill: Cardiovascular System.

5. B. When there is a negative sign next to the blood group type, the Rh factor is not expressed on the surface of the red blood cell. Skill: Cardiovascular System.

6. C. The reduction of melatonin can result in the inability to sleep. Skill: Endocrine System.

7. B. Neuromodulators and neurotransmitters are secreted by nerve cells and aid the nervous system. As an example, acetylcholine is produced during stressful encounters. Skill: Endocrine System.

8. D. The pancreas secretes digestive enzymes into the small intestine. Skill: Gastrointestinal System.

9. A. Food does not pass through the liver, gallbladder, or pancreas. Skill: Gastrointestinal System.

10. A. The correct sequence of the three parts of the small intestine is duodenum → jejunum → ileum. **Skill: Gastrointestinal System.**

11. D. The stratum spinosum contains keratinocytes, which are affected by squamous cell carcinoma. This skin layer is part of the epidermis. **Skill: Integumentary System.**

12. A. Wrinkly skin due to aging occurs because the epidermis is thinning. Typically, aging slows down physiological processes like cell division. Improving this process to generate new cells may help thicken the epidermis and slow down the effects of aging, such as the appearance of wrinkles. **Skill: Integumentary System.**

13. B. At the site of injury or damage to a blood vessel, platelets help repair the damaged area. **Skill: Cardiovascular System.**

14. C. The bloodstream of the vaccinated person contains memory cells that are directed against a specific pathogen. **Skill: The Lymphatic System.**

15. B. Myosin heads attach to thin actin filaments to form crossbridges. These attachments can only form when the myosin head is energized with ATP. **Skill: Muscular System.**

16. A. According to the slide filament theory, after a myosin head attaches to actin it forms a crossbridge. Because of this crossbridge, myosin can pull actin closer to the M-line. **Skill: Muscular System.**

17. B. The outermost layer of connective tissue in skeletal muscle, the epimysium is dense and protects the skeletal muscle from friction when it rubs against other muscles or bones. It also groups all fascicles, or bundles of muscle fibers, together to form a skeletal muscle. **Skill: Muscular System.**

18. C. Individual bones connect at joints. Joints help bones move, and the degree of movement depends on the type of joint. Of the three types of joints, synovial joints offer the largest freedom of movement. This is because the bones are separated by a joint cavity. **Skill: Muscular System.**

19. A. If a presynaptic neuron forms a synapse with the postsynaptic membrane of a gland, and a neurotransmitter binds to receptors on a gland, this will stimulate a release of hormones from that gland. **Skill: The Nervous System.**

20. D. Neuroglia provide protection and support for neurons. They do not participate in the generation of a neural impulse, which means they are unable to transmit electric signals or generate action potentials. **Skill: The Nervous System.**

21. A. After a neuron is stimulated and an action potential travels down the axon, sodium ions flood the axon terminal bulb of the presynaptic membrane. This triggers calcium ions to flood the axon bulb, causing vesicles that carry neurotransmitters to contract and move closer to the presynaptic membrane. **Skill: The Nervous System.**

22. B. Menopause is caused by age-related, fundamental hormonal changes in the female body. It marks the end of the regular menstrual cycle. The age of menopause varies widely, but it usually occurs from the mid-40s to the mid-50s, with the average age in the United States being about 51. **Skill: Reproductive System.**

23. B. The muscular uterus is primarily responsible for pushing the baby out of the mother's body. **Skill: Reproductive System.**

24. A. Although the respiratory system ensures blood contains enough oxygen to be delivered to cells in the body, the cardiovascular system plays a direct role in supplying that oxygen to the cells. **Skill: The Respiratory System.**

25. C. During internal respiration, gas exchange occurs between blood and tissues of the body. Red blood cells exchange oxygen for carbon dioxide. **Skill: The Respiratory System.**

26. B. The diaphragm is a dome-shaped muscle that flattens when a person inhales. **Skill: The Respiratory System.**

27. B. Compact bone is a dense type of bone tissue that is comprised of units called osteons. It provides the hard, outer surface of bone and creates a tough protective layer around the soft, spongy bone. **Skill: Skeletal System.**

28. B. Osteons are small units found inside compact bone. Compact bone is the outer surface of bone that is surrounded by the periosteum. **Skill: Skeletal System.**

29. C. Inside the medullary cavity is yellow marrow and red marrow. Yellow marrow consists primarily of fat cells, while red morrow is the site of hematopoiesis, or formation of red blood cells. **Skill: Skeletal System.**

30. C. There are two sphincters in the urinary system, one at the beginning of bladder and the other at the end of the bladder. The sphincter at the end of the bladder pushes urine to the urethra, where it can be excreted. This sphincter is under voluntary control. **Skill: The Urinary System.**

31. D. The skeletal system serves many purposes, includingproviding support. Bones and cartilage help maintain body posture and comprise the framework of the skeletal system. **Skill: Skeletal System.**

32. B. Both the distal convoluted tubule and collecting ducts are permeable to water when ADH is present. This means water is steadily reabsorbed and retained, causing the volume of urine that is excreted to decrease. Urine concentration increases. **Skill: The Urinary System.**

33. D. Both the electron transport chain and oxidative phosphorylation are major energy producers during cellular respiration. Collectively, these metabolic pathways produce upwards of 32 ATP per glucose molecule. **Skill: An Introduction to Biology.**

34. A. The control variable is a standard or constant that is used for comparisons. **Skill: An Introduction to Biology.**

35. D. Monosaccharides are monomers used to create larger molecules called carbohydrates. **Skill: An Introduction to Biology.**

36. B. Lipid synthesis is anabolic because monomers like fatty acids are used to synthesize lipid molecules. **Skill: An Introduction to Biology.**

37. A. Organisms are classified as either autotrophs or heterotrophs according to how they obtain energy. Autotrophs obtain energy through sunlight, whereas heterotrophs obtain energy through food. **Skill: Cell Structure, Function, and Type.**

38. B. Heterotrophs such as bears are organisms that function as consumers and ingest food as an energy source. **Skill: Cell Structure, Function, and Type.**

39. A. Prokaryotes like bacteria participate in asexual reproduction. This means they can create offspring using a single parent. **Skill: Cellular Reproduction, Cellular Respiration, and Photosynthesis.**

40. C. There are three phases that occur before a cell reaches the mitotic phase: G1, synthesis, G2 phase. A molecule of DNA doubles during the synthesis phase before beginning to prepare for cell division during G2. **Skill: Cellular Reproduction, Cellular Respiration, and Photosynthesis.**

41. D. When two sister chromatids come together, they are bound by a centromere; this enables them to form a loosely condensed chromosome. **Skill: Cellular Reproduction, Cellular Respiration, and Photosynthesis.**

42. A. A DNA molecule and its associated proteins coil tightly right before cellular division. **Skill: Genetics and DNA.**

43. C. Transcription manufactures ribonucleic acid (RNA). **Skill: Genetics and DNA.**

44. A. The theory of heredity includes the idea that an individual receives one allele from each parent. In doing so, this increases the potential for genetic diversity within a given population. Phenotype determines the physical appearance of a person and all of these traits come from both parents. **Skill: Genetics and DNA.**

45. A. A single DNA molecule is packaged in a rod-shaped structure also known as a chromosome. **Skill: Genetics and DNA.**

46. D. During sublimation, a solid turns into a gas. Because solids have less energy than gases, the solid will have to absorb energy to undergo this phase change. **Skill: States of Matter.**

47. B. The graph shows a non-correlation between height and birth month. This means birth month has no effect on how tall the baby will be. **Skill: Designing an Experiment.**

48. C. The atomic number of an element is determined by its number of protons. Lithium has an atomic number of 3, which means that if an atom has 3 protons, it is an atom of lithium. **Skill: Scientific Notation.**

49. C. Zinc-64 contains 30 protons and 34 neutrons. An isotope would contain the same number of protons but a different number of neutrons. **Skill: Scientific Notation.**

50. C. Families in the periodic table are associated with groups (columns). Strontium is the only element listed that is in group 2 with calcium. **Skill: Scientific Notation.**

51. B. Fluorine and bromine are the only pair located in the same group (column) of the periodic table, group 17. **Skill: Scientific Notation.**

52. C. Intensive properties do not depend on the amount of matter that is present. Intensive properties do not change according to conditions. **Skill: Properties of Matter.**

53. C. Melting is a phase change of a solid to a liquid. **Skill: Properties of Matter.**

Section IV. English and Language Usage

1. D. They used to live in the Pacific Northwest. Specific geographic regions are capitalized. **Skill: Capitalization.**

2. C. *No, I am not leaving yet.* Commas are used after yes or no. **Skill: Punctuation.**

3. B. With words ending in -z, add -es. **Skill: Spelling.**

4. A. *Knives* is the plural form of knife. *Salmon* is a non-count noun, so it does not have a plural form. **Skill: Nouns.**

5. A. *Him* is an object pronoun. **Skill: Pronouns.**

6. B. *Founding* is an adjective that describes the noun *fathers.* **Skill: Adjectives and Adverbs.**

7. D. *From, to,* and *for* are prepositions. **Skill: Conjunctions and Prepositions.**

8. A. This is a past tense negative, so it takes the helping verb *did* with the base form *like.* **Skill: Verbs and Verb Tenses.**

9. B. *He* is third person singular. **Skill: Subject and Verb Agreement.**

10. B. With *neither/nor,* if both subjects are third person singular, the verb should take the third person singular form. **Skill: Subject and Verb Agreement.**

11. C. The verb *honor* must agree with the subject *Americans.* **Skill: Subject and Verb Agreement.**

12. C. *But.* It is the only conjunction that fits within the context of the sentence. **Skill: Types of Clauses.**

13. D. Independent clause. The sentence has a subject and a verb and expresses a complete thought. **Skill: Types of Clauses.**

14. B. This sentence correctly fixes the fragment. **Skill: Types of Sentences.**

15. A. This option would make the sentence a simple sentence. **Skill: Types of Sentences.**

16. A. *Broadens their perspective* would be parallel in structure to the other items since they are longer phrases and use the same verb form. **Skill: Types of Sentences.**

17. B. A birthday party. It is an informal setting with friends and family. **Skill: Formal and Informal Language.**

18. A. This essay claims that sugar is bad for people. In academic writing, pronouns such as *I* should not be used. **Skill: Formal and Informal Language.**

19. C. The meaning of stall in this context is "to stop running." The phrase "stop working" helps you figure out which meaning of stall is being used. **Skill: Context Clues and Multiple Meaning Words.**

20. C. The meaning of apathetic in this context is "indifferent or unconcerned." The word "nonchalantly" helps you figure out the meaning of apathetic. **Skill: Context Clues and Multiple Meaning Words.**

21. B. The word "staple" has more than one meaning. **Skill: Context Clues and Multiple Meaning Words.**

22. B. The meaning of produce in the context of this sentence is "manufacture or build." **Skill: Context Clues and Multiple Meaning Words.**

23. D. The meaning of advocate in the context of this sentence is "supporter." **Skill: Context Clues and Multiple Meaning Words.**

24. C. The root word *nat* means "born," so *natal* means "relating to birth." **Skill: Root Words, Prefixes, and Suffixes.**

25. C. The root that means "sound" is *phon* as in the word *microphone.* **Skill: Root Words, Prefixes, and Suffixes.**

26. D. The prefix that means "after" is *post-* as in the word *posthumously.* **Skill: Root Words, Prefixes, and Suffixes.**

27. A. The prefix *poly-* means "many" and the root word "the" means "god," so a polytheistic religion would be a religion in which its people believe in many gods. **Skill: Root Words, Prefixes, and Suffixes.**

28. B. The root word *spher* means "ball-like," so *spherical* means "round." **Skill: Root Words, Prefixes, and Suffixes.**

TEAS Practice Exam 6

Section I. Reading

You have 64 minutes to complete 53 questions.

Read the following sentence and answer questions 1-3.

Studies conducted on numerous kindergarten programs across the country have revealed eye-opening evidence that today's kindergarten curriculum looks more like the curriculum taught in first grade classrooms thirty years ago.

1. **What is the main idea of the above sentence?**

   A. What kindergarten is

   B. How kindergarten has changed

   C. What students learn in kindergarten

   D. What the kindergarten curriculum is

2. **Imagine this sentence is a *supporting detail* in a well-developed paragraph. Which of the following sentences would best function as a *topic sentence*?**

   A. The curriculum seen in today's kindergarten classrooms may not be developmentally appropriate for children.

   B. Teaching styles have changed dramatically over the course of the last thirty years.

   C. Play-based learning is still a big part of today's kindergarten classrooms.

   D. Studies have shown that national-based standards lead to more success in the classroom.

3. Imagine this sentence is the *topic sentence* of a well-developed paragraph. Which of the following sentences would best function as a *supporting detail*?

   A. Some students enter kindergarten with a rich nursery school experience while others enter the school environment for the first time in their lives.

   B. Kindergarten is a German word that literally means "a garden for children."

   C. While kindergarteners from years ago only needed to begin to learn basic concepts of print in reading, today's kindergarteners are expected to be at an E reading level when leaving the classroom.

   D. Kindergarten is the time when children acquire the necessary early educational skills to prepare them to be full-fledged students who are ready for first grade.

4. A summary is a_____.

   A. retelling of all the ideas of a text

   B. review of the final idea of a text

   C. rundown of the first idea of a text

   D. restatement of the main ideas of a text

5. Which graphic would best support a paragraph about the different parts of a car engine and their functions?

A. Diagram   C. Bar graph

B. Flowchart   D. Pie chart

6. Which graphic would best support a paragraph explaining the percentage breakdowns of how a charity organization plans to spend a large donation?

A. Diagram   C. Bar graph

B. Flowchart   D. Pie chart

Study the outline below and answer questions 7-11.

I. Introduction - We need more racial and gender diversity in our superheroes.

II. The lack of diversity in comics means kids get the message that only white males can be heroic.

    A. Quote from Sid Markell (pg. 213): "When I was a kid, imagining myself saving the world meant imagining I was white."

    B. Quote from Lydia Green (kenswicktimes.com): "I remember people seeing my comments and saying, 'You like reading *that*?' I heard, 'You think you can be *important*?'"

    C. Markell and Green aren't just interacting with superhero comics as fiction; they're seeing them as messages from a real world that excludes them.

III. Conclusion

    A. Recap main points.

    B. Let's create a world where all kids are invited to imagine they can be heroes.

7. Which statement from the outline will be the main idea of the essay?

A. We need more racial and gender diversity in our superheroes.

B. Kids get the message that only white males can be heroic.

C. Markell and Green aren't just interacting with superhero comics as fiction.

D. Let's create a world where all kids are invited to imagine they can be heroes.

8. What does the writer of this outline still need to do?

A. Collect evidence to back up the main idea

B. Figure out how to end the essay

C. Create an attention-grabbing opening statement

D. Decide how to organize the ideas in the essay

9. The writer of this outline wants to add this sentence:

This world needs all the heroes it can get.

Where would it fit best?

A. In the introduction, before the thesis statement

B. In the introduction, after the thesis statement

C. In the body, before the topic sentence

D. In the body, after the first quotation

10. **The writer of this outline wants to add a second body paragraph. Which statement could function as a topic sentence that clearly adds new information to support the main idea?**

   A. Girls and women tend to gravitate away from careers our society associates with heroic actions.

   B. Green writes, "As a kid I wanted to be a firefighter, but people always laughed at me when I said so."

   C. If our fiction presented more women and people of color as superheroes, more kids would likely grow up aspiring to save others.

   D. Superhero characters in comics and the movies are almost all white and male, sending fans the message that these traits are necessary for heroism.

11. **The information in parentheses under II.A. and II.B. is most likely:**

   A. a visual element the writer wants to add while drafting.

   B. intended to remind the writer to look up different quotations.

   C. source information the writer will later use to create citations.

   D. an error that will need to be fixed at a later stage in the writing process.

12. **Which of the following is *not* a form of prewriting?**

   A. Revising

   B. Outlining

   C. Brainstorming

   D. Mind mapping

Read the following sentence and answer questions 13-14.

   The archeologists uncovered many fascinating objects at their dig site.

13. **Which word could replace *objects* above to give the sentence more precise word choice without changing the meaning?**

   A. Bodies

   B. Things

   C. Artifacts

   D. Phenomena

14. **It would likely be a poor choice to use *artifacts* as a more precise replacement for *objects* in the sentence above when addressing an audience of:**

   A. fifth graders.

   B. archeologists.

   C. history teachers.

   D. science journalists.

15. **An essay has _____ if the ideas are logical and consistent.**

   A. effect

   B. rhetoric

   C. coherence

   D. organization

16. **Read the following sentences:**

   Our understanding of paleontology continues to grow and change. Until recently, we believed all dinosaurs had died out at the end of the Cretaceous Period 65 million years ago. We now understand that one group of dinosaurs survived and evolved into birds.

   Which words and phrases are transitions?

   A. Until recently; we

   B. Until recently; now

   C. All; we

   D. All; now

7. Read the following sentences:

<u>Due to the fact that</u> fatty pork is often cured and turned into unhealthy products like bacon, many health-conscious consumers fail to recognize the potential of pork. <u>On the other hand</u>, lean and unprocessed pork products can be a valuable part of a healthy diet.

Which transitions could replace the wordy phrases underlined and improve the writing style without changing the meaning?

A. First; likewise

B. Then; moreover

C. Because; however

D. For example; consequently

Read the following passage and answer questions 18-23.

When Dr. Kingston Hussein saw an announcement for a conference titled Ethics of Human

Embryonic Research, he booked his tickets six months in advance.

"We need to stop and reflect on the ramifications of every new development in our research," said Dr. Hussein, the lead researcher in embryology at the Dampson Crockett Institute in Lewiston, Maine. "Every researcher in our field feels the weight of responsibility here. It's what we talk about when we go out for drinks after work."

Attitudes like Dr. Hussein's stand in stark contrast to common public perceptions of embryonic research. "These guys think they're gods," said Liz Goode, chairwoman of The Center for Ethical and Dignified Humanity, an organization that opposes all research on human embryos. "They want to get rich selling designer babies to billionaires. It's a nightmare."

An outside observer might expect a researcher like Dr. Hussein to avoid all contact with an activist like Goode. On the contrary, Dr. Hussein wrote to the organizers of the conference and requested that they invite Goode to host a panel. "We need dialogue," he said. "We need to hear what makes the public uncomfortable." He chuckled. "We also need to inform them about what we're actually doing."

And what *are* embryonic researchers doing? "Not building designer babies," he said. Dr. Hussein uses words like "run-of-the-mill medical" to describe his research goals. For instance, he is seeking causes and treatments for a variety of neurological disorders.

18. Which adjective most accurately describes the author's tone?

A. Scathing   C. Negative

B. Objective   D. Ironic

19. Reread the following quotation from the passage:

"Every researcher in our field feels the weight of responsibility here. It's what we talk about when we go out for drinks after work."

Which adjective most accurately describes Dr. Hussein's tone?

A. Scathing   C. Earnest

B. Apathetic   D. Ironic

20. Reread the following quotation from the passage:

"These guys think they're gods...They want to get rich selling designer babies to billionaires. It's a nightmare."

Which adjective most accurately describes Liz Goode's tone?

A. Harsh   C. Earnest

B. Tolerant   D. Ironic

21. **Which phrase functions as a transition to juxtapose dissimilar ideas in the passage?**

A. Attitudes like Dr. Hussein's

B. For instance

C. An outside observer

D. On the contrary

22. **Which phrase functions as a transition to introduce an example in the passage?**

A. Attitudes like Dr. Hussein's

B. For instance

C. An outside observer

D. On the contrary

23. Reread the following sentences from the passage:

"We need dialogue," he said. "We need to hear what makes the public uncomfortable." He chuckled. "We also need to inform them about what we're actually doing."

Which word or phrase functions as a transition in these sentences?

A. He said   C. Also

B. He chuckled   D. Actually

24. **Read the sentences below.**

Meredith shows clearly that she is driven to succeed as a gymnast. _____ I have often noticed her waiting outside the gym before it opens at 7:00 a.m. _____ her coaches report that she frequently asks for help with her tumbling skills.

Which words or phrases should be inserted into the blanks to provide clear transitions between these ideas?

A. In conclusion; Thus

B. First; Consequently

C. Although; In contrast

D. For instance; Furthermore

25. **Read the sentences below.**

My pet boa constrictor is not a danger to humans. Despite his size and alarming appearance, he is basically a big, cuddly garden snake.

What is the function of the underlined transition word in sentence two?

A. To express a contrast

B. To provide an example

C. To add emphasis to a point

D. To indicate time or sequence

26. **What is the most likely purpose of an article explaining why Eastern medicine is better than Western medicine?**

A. To decide   C. To persuade

B. To inform   D. To entertain

27. **What is the most likely purpose of a realistic fiction book about one family's experience living in a foreign country?**

A. To decide   C. To persuade

B. To inform   D. To entertain

Read the following text and answer questions 28-30.

As Time Goes On is a painfully realistic depiction of what life is like for some senior citizens in the twilight of their lives. Tabitha Reynolds artfully captures the harsh reality people face when they grow old. From one's physical limitations to the emotional toll of letting go of one's former self, Reynolds pays homage to this fragile yet meaningful time in a person's life.

The book chronicles the final years of Audrey Lacoste's life. A former prima ballerina, Audrey is now a prisoner to her rheumatoid arthritis. The disease has limited Audrey's body in ways she could never have imagined. Her physical ailment coupled with the loss of her beloved husband causes her two self-involved children to move her into Sunshine Cove, an assisted living facility. The facility is anything but sunny, but slowly the light in Audrey's life begins to flicker once again when she makes an unexpected friend.

A *New York Times* best seller for seven consecutive weeks, *As Time Goes On* is a must read. The words will make you laugh, cry, gasp and sigh as you travel along the rocky road to the end of Audrey's life.

28. The purpose of this passage is to:

A. decide.   C. persuade.

B. inform.   D. entertain.

29. Which detail from the passage is factual?

A. *As Time Goes On* is a painfully realistic depiction of what life is like for some senior citizens...

B. Tabitha Reynolds artfully captures the harsh reality people face as they grow old.

C. The book chronicles the final years of Audrey Lacoste's life.

D. ...*As Time Goes On* is a must read.

30. The author of the passage includes details about Audrey Lacoste's life in order to appeal to the reader's:

A. reason.   C. feelings.

B. trust.   D. knowledge.

Read the map below and answer questions 31-35.

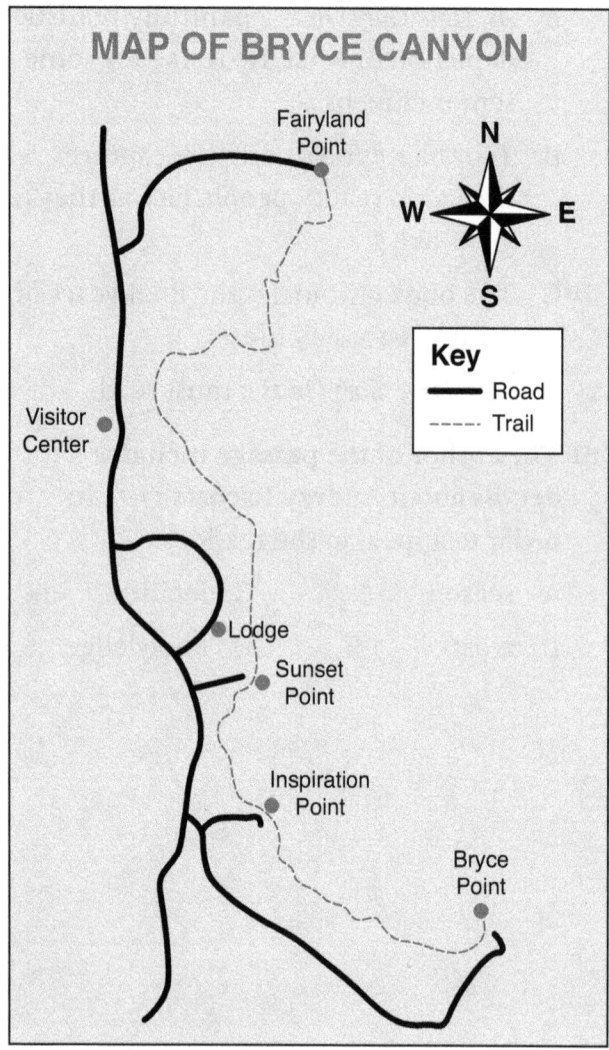

MAP OF BRYCE CANYON

Fairland Point

N
W   E
S

Visitor Center

Key
——— Road
- - - - Trail

Lodge
Sunset Point

Inspiration Point

Bryce Point

31. A person could get from the Lodge to Fairyland Point by:

A. driving east on the road.

B. driving west on the road.

C. walking north on the Rim Trail.

D. walking south on the Rim Trail.

32. Which feature on the map is between Sunset Point and Bryce Point?

A. Sunrise Point

B. Fairyland Point

C. Visitor's Center

D. Inspiration Point

33. How could a person travel from the Visitor's Center to Bryce Point without touching Sunset Point?

A. By keeping to the main road

B. By walking along the Rim Trail

C. By taking the route to Fairyland Point

D. By driving the loop road near the Lodge

34. Which feature on the map is farthest west?

A. Bryce Point

B. Sunrise Point

C. Fairyland Point

D. Visitor's Center

35. The legend shows:

A. how to differentiate between a road and a trail.

B. where visitors can leave a parked vehicle while hiking.

C. which point is the Visitor's Center and which is the Lodge.

D. how to see all the viewpoints in Bryce Canyon on a single visit.

36. Carla is trying to limit her calorie intake. When she buys a bottle of soda, she is pleased to see a low value of 100 calories per serving. Before she pours herself a glass, she should check the number of:

A. servings per bottle.

B. calories per gram of fat.

C. calories per gram of sugar.

D. servings in a glass of water.

37. If you are using a book for research but it contains more information than you need, which text feature is most likely to help you find the most important pages to read?

A. Index

C. Sidebars

B. Italics

D. Endnotes

38. Which of the following is an opinion?

A. Doctors should offer holistic approaches instead of relying solely on medication.

B. Non-steroidal anti-inflammatory drugs are the most prescribed medications by doctors.

C. Pharmaceutical companies spend double the amount on marketing to doctors than they spend on research.

D. A 2018 study predicts that the U.S. will experience a shortage of between 42,600 and 121,300 physicians by 2030.

Read the following passage and answer questions 39-44.

Most people under age 35 spend too much time on social media. Statistics show that over nine out of ten teens go online using a mobile device daily, and seven out of ten use more than one major social media site. This is too much. Teens and young adults must limit their use of social media or face deteriorating relationships in real life. You know how frustrating it feels to try to talk to someone who constantly disengages to check a phone. Interacting online can be fun, but it never provides as much satisfaction as talking with actual human beings. Social media shouldn't be the primary social outlet for young people because people who rely mainly on the Internet for social interaction are unhappy and unfulfilled.

39. What is the primary argument in the passage?

A. All young people face emotional and social problems.

B. Teens and young adults should limit their social media use.

C. People under age 35 have never known life without the Internet.

D. Disengaging to check a phone can damage real-life social interactions.

40. Which excerpt from the text, if true, is a fact?

A. Most people under age 35 spend too much time on social media.

B. Statistics show that over nine out of ten teens go online using a mobile device daily.

C. Teens and young adults must limit their use of social media or face deteriorating relationships in real life.

D. Interacting online can be fun, but it never provides as much satisfaction as talking with actual human beings.

41. Re-read the following sentence from the passage:

Teens and young adults must limit their use of social media or face deteriorating relationships in real life.

What type of faulty reasoning does this sentence display?

A. Either/or fallacy

B. Circular reasoning

C. Bandwagon argument

D. False statement of cause and effect

42. Re-read the following sentence from the passage:

Interacting online can be fun, but it never provides as much satisfaction as talking with actual human beings.

The reasoning in this sentence is faulty because it makes a(n):

A. circular statement.

B. overgeneralization.

C. bandwagon argument.

D. false statement of cause and effect.

43. Re-read the following sentence from the passage:

Social media shouldn't be the primary social outlet for young people because people who rely mainly on the Internet for social interaction are unhappy and unfulfilled.

The reasoning in this sentence is faulty because it:

A. suggests that an idea is good because everyone is doing it.

B. claims that there are only two ways to solve a complex problem.

C. restates the argument in different words instead of providing evidence.

D. assumes that people socialize because they want to feel happy and fulfilled.

44. Re-read the following sentence from the passage:

Most people under age 35 spend too much time on social media.

This sentence is an opinion because it:

A. reflects a belief, not a verifiable fact.

B. does not say how much is too much.

C. restricts its statement to people under 35.

D. lumps all people under 35 into one category.

Read the following passage and answer questions 45-48.

Adelia stood on the porch in her bathrobe.

"Mr. Snuggles?" she called. "Mr. Snuggles! Come on in, you little vermin."

She peered up and down the street. Sighing, she went back inside and, a moment later, emerged with a metal bowl and a spoon. She rapped on the bowl several times.

"Mr. Snuggles? Breakfast!"

When Mr. Snuggles did not appear, Adelia reached inside and grabbed some keys off a low table. Cinching her bathrobe tightly around her waist, she climbed into the car.

"It's not like I have anything better to do than look for you again," she said.

45. From the text above, you can infer that Adelia is:

A. looking for a pet.

B. calling her son home.

C. a kindhearted person.

D. unconcerned for Mr. Snuggles.

46. Which detail does not provide evidence to back up the conclusion that Adelia is feeling frustrated?

A. She calls Mr. Snuggles "you little vermin."

B. She has not yet gotten dressed for the day.

C. She complains about having to search for Mr. Snuggles.

D. She sighs when Mr. Snuggles does not immediately appear.

47. Which detail from the text supports the inference that Adelia cares what happens to Mr. Snuggles, even if she is angry at him?

A. She goes out to look for him.

B. She keeps her car keys near the door.

C. She is joking when she calls him "vermin."

D. She says she wants to be doing something else.

48. Which sentence of dialogue, if added to the passage, would support the conclusion that Mr. Snuggles actually belongs to someone else?

A. "What ever possessed me to adopt a cat?"

B. "You shed on my sheets, you pee on my couch, and now *this*."

C. "Next time Raul goes out of town, I'm going to babysit his plants instead."

D. "If you make me late again, I'm going to lose my job. Then how will we eat?"

49. **Which of the following is a secondary source?**

    A. The diary of Anne Frank

    B. A biography of Anne Frank

    C. A study guide on the diary of Anne Frank

    D. An encyclopedia article about Anne Frank

50. **Which of the following could not be a primary source?**

    A. An oil painting

    B. A personal email

    C. An autobiography

    D. An encyclopedia entry

Read the following text and answer questions 51-53.

When my mother was a teenager, most kids didn't have cell phones. If she wanted to talk to her friends after school, she had to call their landline. Sometimes a friend's mom or dad answered, and she had to ask to talk to their kid. She says that was awkward. Also, if she and a friend talked on the phone for a long time, the whole family's phone line was busy, so nobody else could get calls. Parents got mad at kids for tying up the phone too long.

Today, every kid I know has a smartphone. We talk and text whenever we want, and none of us ever have awkward conversations with our friends' parents. But in some ways, parents today have more control. A lot of parents check kids' phone records and read their texts, so they can tell if their kids are up to no good. Families don't all rely on one phone line, so when kids talk for a long time, we don't prevent anyone else in the family from communicating with their friends. But parents today still get mad—mainly because kids' phone habits cost too much money.

51. **What category of writing is this?**

    A. Narrative   C. Expository

    B. Technical   D. Persuasive

52. **The structure of the passage is:**

    A. description.

    B. cause/effect.

    C. problem-solution.

    D. compare/contrast.

53. **What is the genre of the passage?**

    A. Essay

    B. Criticism

    C. Biography

    D. Autobiography

SECTION II. MATHEMATICS

You will have 54 minutes to complete 36 questions.

. Elementary school students were surveyed about their favorite animals at a zoo. The circle graph shows the results. Which statement is true for the circle graph?

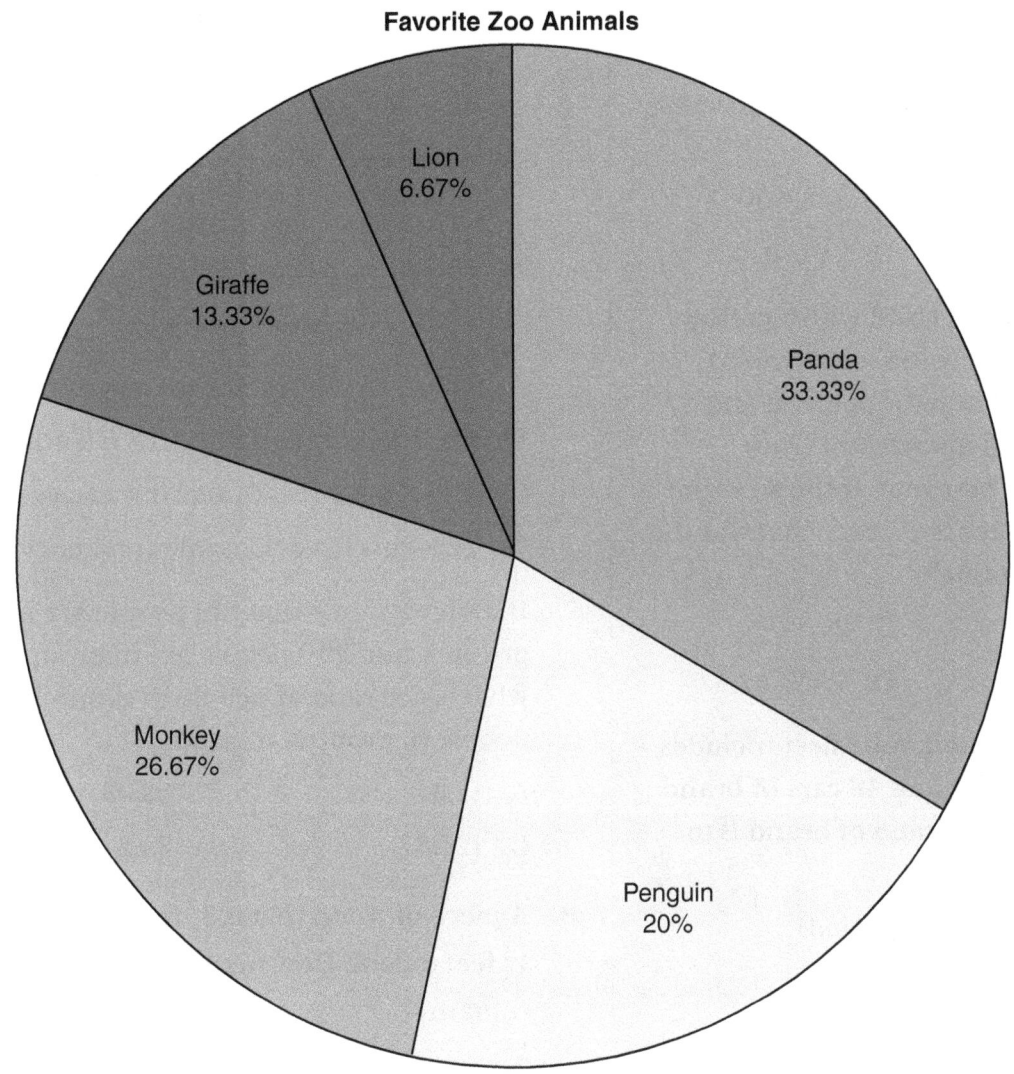

Favorite Zoo Animals

A. The penguins were the second-favorite animals.

B. No group of animals makes up one-third of the graph.

C. Sixty percent of the students like pandas and monkeys.

D. Fifty percent of the students like giraffes, lions, and penguins.

2. Find the difference.

$2\frac{2}{3}-\frac{1}{6}$

A. $2\frac{1}{3}$ C. $2\frac{1}{2}$

B. $1\frac{2}{3}$ D. $1\frac{1}{3}$

3. A family pays 18% the value of a home as the down payment. If they paid $63,000 as their down payment, what is the value of the home they purchased?

A. $113,400   C. $98,000

B. $350,000   D. $176,400

4. A father sets up his child with a college savings account. He makes an initial deposit of $500 into the account and earns a tremendous amount from interest for the first year. If the account has $712 in it after one year, what was the annual interest rate?

A. 14.24%   C. 24.4%

B. 23.5%   D. 42.4%

5. If a company's automobile fleet includes 132 cars of brand A and 48 cars of brand B, what is the fleet's ratio of brand B to brand A?

A. 4:11   C. 15:11

B. 11:15   D. 11:4

6. The histogram below shows the number of text messages between a group of friends in a week. Which statement is true for the histogram?

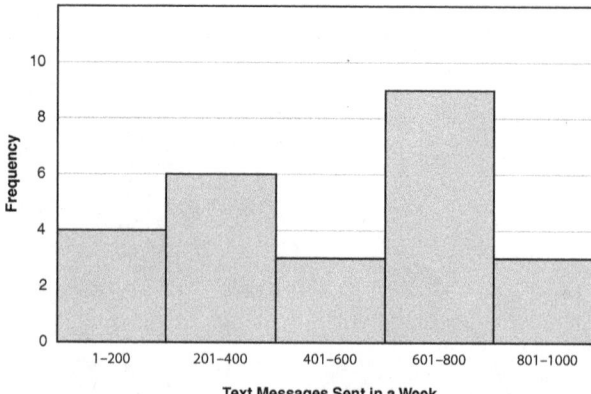

A. There are 30 friends in the group.

B. The highest frequency is 8 friends.

C. The bin size is 1,000 text messages.

D. Two bins have the same frequency.

7. If a survey finds that 120 people are in group X and 230 people are in group Y, what is the ratio of people in group Y to people in group X or group Y?

A. 12:35   C. 23:35

B. 12:23   D. 35:23

8. A piece of wood that is $5\frac{2}{3}$ feet long has $1\frac{1}{4}$ feet cut off. How many feet of wood remain?

A. $4\frac{1}{12}$ C. $6\frac{1}{12}$

B. $4\frac{5}{12}$ D. $6\frac{5}{12}$

9. Which proportion yields a number for the unknown that is different from the others?

A. $\frac{13}{75}=\frac{158}{?}$ C. $\frac{158}{?}=\frac{13}{75}$

B. $\frac{75}{13}=\frac{?}{158}$ D. $\frac{75}{13}=\frac{158}{?}$

0. The box plot below shows the winning margin of two basketball teams during the season. Select the true statement about the interquartile range.

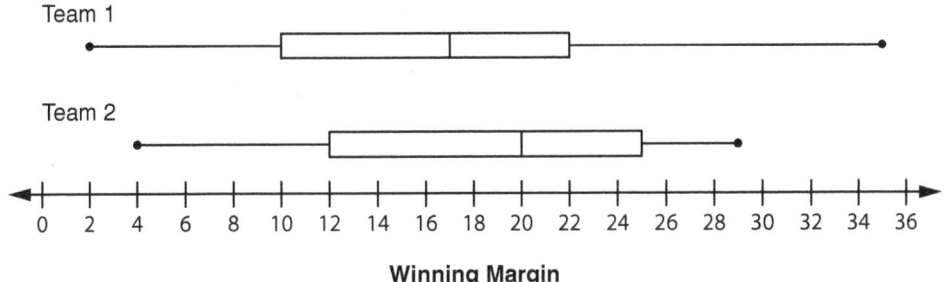

A. The interquartile range is greater for Team 2 by 1 point.

B. The interquartile range is greater for Team 2 by 3 points.

C. The interquartile range is greater for Team 1 by 6 points.

D. The interquartile range is greater for Team 1 by 8 points.

1. Apply the polynomial identity to rewrite the expression.

$16x^2-121$

A. $(x + 11)(x-11)$

C. $(4x + 11)(4x-11)$

B. $(x-11)^2$

D. $(4x-11)^2$

12. Change $7\frac{13}{20}$ to a decimal. Simplify completely.

A. 7.55

C. 7.65

B. 7.6

D. 7.7

12. If a tree grows an average of 4.2 inches in a day, what is the rate of change in its height per month? Assume a month is 30 days.

A. 0.14 inches per month

C. 34.2 inches per month

B. 4.2 inches per month

D. 126 inches per month

14. Write 290% as a fraction.

A. $2\frac{9}{200}$

C. $2\frac{9}{20}$

B. $2\frac{9}{100}$

D. $2\frac{9}{10}$

15. Convert 147 liters to kiloliters. (Note: 1 kiloliter is equal to 1000 liters).

A. 0.147 kiloliters

C. 1,470 kiloliters

B. 1.47 kiloliters

D. 147,000 kiloliters

16. A student athlete gets out of practice at 4:00PM and needs to get to work that is 15 miles away by 4:30PM. He wants 10 minutes to change into his uniform, so he needs to figure out how fast to drive. On average, how fast does he need to travel?

A. 45 mph

C. 54 mph

B. 60 mph

D. 62 mph

17. Solve the equation for the unknown.

$\frac{x}{2} + 5 = 8$

A. $\frac{3}{2}$

C. 6

B. $\frac{5}{2}$

D. 26

18. Multiply $\frac{2}{5} \times 3$.

A. $\frac{2}{15}$

C. $2\frac{3}{5}$

B. $1\frac{1}{5}$

D. $3\frac{2}{5}$

19. The table shows the expenses and revenue for the first six months of a year in millions of dollars. Select the correct bar graph for this data.

Month	January	February	March	April	May	June
Revenue	5	4.5	6	6	6.5	7
Expenses	4	5	5.5	6	5	5.5

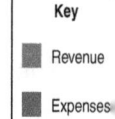
A.
Expenses and Revenue

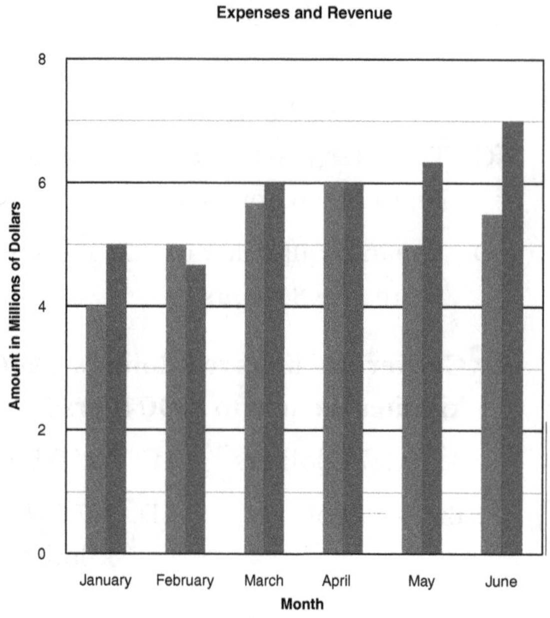

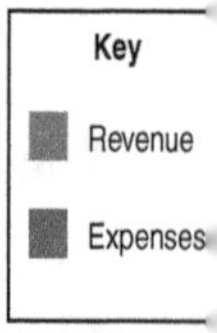

C.
Expenses and Revenue

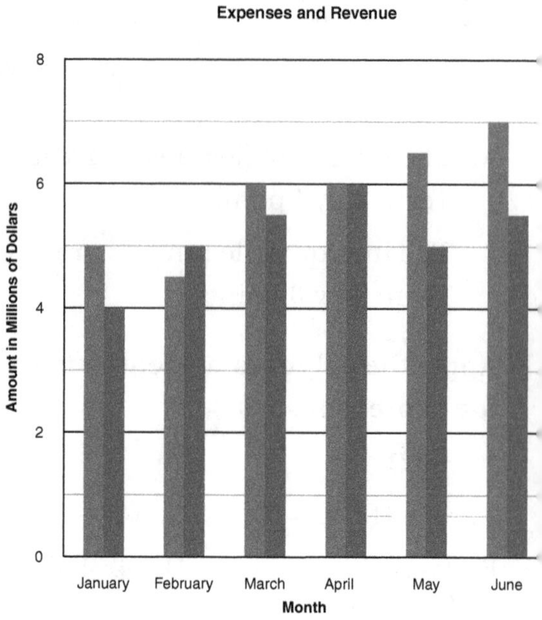

B.
Expenses and Revenue

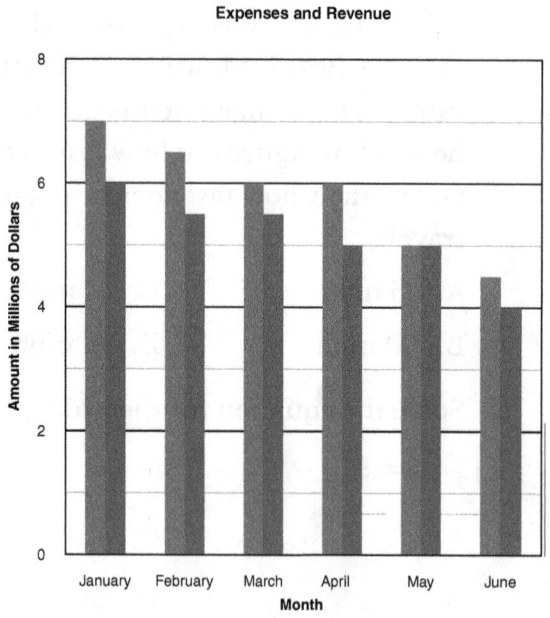

D.
Expenses and Revenue

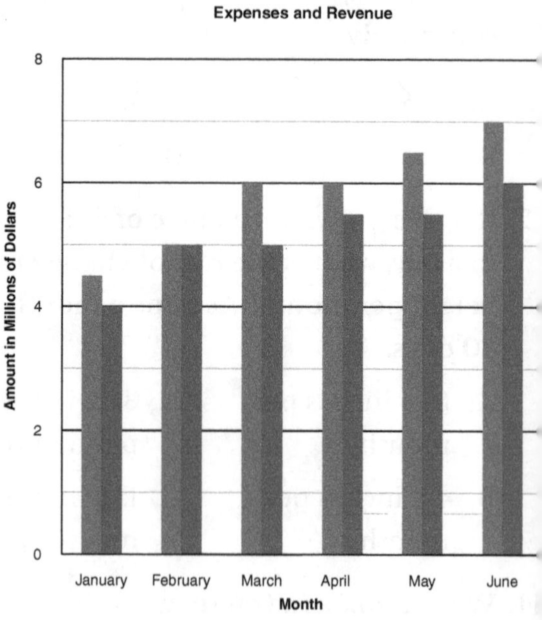

20. A gardener wants to create a border around his garden with small pieces of wood. To make his border, he needs 20 feet of wood, but the planks he likes are only sold in $\frac{1}{2}$ yard pieces. How many pieces of wood does he need to buy?

    A. 7   C. 14

    B. 10   D. 18

21. If a taxi costs $6.00 plus $5.65 per mile and a customer needs to travel 18 miles (*m*), select the correct equation that represents how much the cab fare cost.

    A. 18*m* + $5.65 = $107.70

    C. $6.00*m* + $5.65 = $107.70

    B. $5.65*m* + $6.00 = $107.70

    D. $5.65 + (18 ÷ *m*) = $107.70

22. Eric buys $2\frac{2}{5}$ pounds of apples each week for four weeks. How many total pounds does he buy?

    A. $7\frac{3}{5}$ C. $9\frac{3}{5}$

    B. $8\frac{2}{5}$ D. $10\frac{2}{5}$

23. Solve for the value of y when x = 3.

    $y = (x^3 + 5) \div 4$

    A. 3   C. 7

    B. 8   D. 4

24. A nurse earns $21 an hour and 114% of her hourly rate for overtime. If she works a full 40 hours and 12 hours of overtime, how much will her paycheck for the week be?

    A. $1,092.00   C. $287.28

    B. $840.00   D. $1,127.28

25. $\frac{3}{14} \div 3$

    A. $\frac{1}{42}$ C. $\frac{1}{3}$

    B. $\frac{1}{14}$ D. $\frac{9}{14}$

26. A company manager is responsible for paying $\frac{1}{6}$ of the bill for a staff outing, while the rest is paid for with company expense money. If the staff outing bill comes to ta total of $262.52, how much money will the manager have to pay?

    A. $43.75   C. $218.77

    B. $15.75   D. $59.50

27. Find the area in square centimeters of a circle with a diameter of 16 centimeters. Use 3.14 for π

    A. 25.12   C. 100.48

    B. 50.24   D. 200.96

28. Solve the equation for the unknown.

    $\frac{1}{3}(3x + 2) + 3 = 2x + 3$

    A. −4   C. $\frac{2}{3}$

    B. $-\frac{2}{3}$ D. 4

29. A high school closes the track for maintenance, so the track team decides to run around the school buildings for practice. If one lap is equivalent to $\frac{8}{10}$ of a mile, how many laps around the school must the team run to do a workout equal to 4 miles?

    A. 6   C. 5

    B. 3.5   D. 4.5

30. Justin works 34 hours a week at one job and 22 hours a week at another job. Since there are 24 hours in a day, how much of a 7-day week is Justin spending at work?

    A. $\frac{1}{2}$ C. $\frac{1}{3}$

    B. $\frac{3}{5}$ D. $\frac{2}{7}$

31. The circle graph shows the daily activities of a student. Which statement is true for the circle graph?

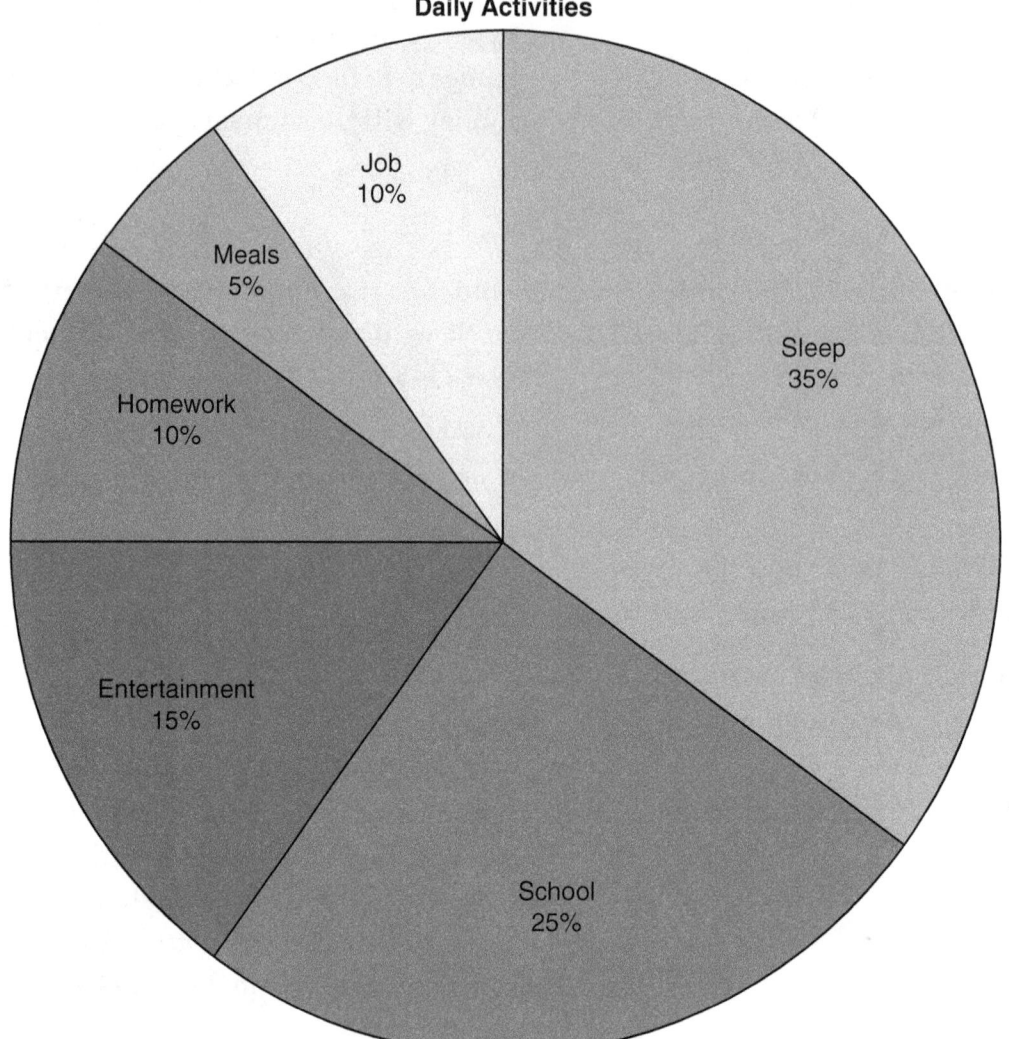

Daily Activities

Job
10%

Meals
5%

Homework
10%

Sleep
35%

Entertainment
15%

School
25%

A. Homework and job take up the least time.

B. The amount of time in school is the largest category.

C. Other categories besides sleep and school are over 50% of the time.

D. Entertainment and homework total is the same as the amount of time in school.

32. Solve for x.

   $(8 - 3)x = 3 \times 5$

   A. 3

   B. 5

   C. 1

   D. 12

33. Convert 1,000 fluid ounces to gallons.

   A. 7.8125 gallons

   B. 15.625 gallons

   C. 31.25 gallons

   D. 62.5 gallons

34. 12°C is what temperature in Fahrenheit?
(Note: $°F = \frac{9}{5}C + 32$)

   A. 24°F   C. 67°F

   B. 54°F   D. 79°F

35. Jayden rides his bike for $2\frac{3}{4}$ miles. He takes a break and rides another $3\frac{1}{3}$ miles. How many miles does he ride?

   A. $5\frac{1}{12}$ C. $6\frac{1}{12}$

   B. $5\frac{4}{7}$ D. $6\frac{4}{7}$

36. A group of friends divide a box of 56 pieces of chalk to draw with on the cement. If one girl takes 8 pieces of chalk, how much of the box did she take?

   A. $\frac{1}{7}$ C. $\frac{1}{10}$

   B. $\frac{1}{5}$ D. $\frac{1}{6}$

SECTION III. SCIENCE

You have 63 minutes to complete 53 questions.

1. **Which feedback mechanism is responsible for a fever?**
   A. Equal
   B. Negative
   C. Neutral
   D. Positive

2. **What are the subdivisions of the dorsal cavity, located in the back of the human body?**
   A. Cranial and spinal
   B. Dorsal and ventral
   C. Lateral and proximal
   D. Inferior and superior

3. **Which anatomical position promotes access to the stomach?**
   A. medial
   B. prone
   C. superficial
   D. supine

4. **Which is the correct order of formed elements in blood from smallest to largest cell size?**
   A. Erythrocytes, thrombocytes, and leukocytes
   B. Thrombocytes, leukocytes, and erythrocytes
   C. Thrombocytes, erythrocytes, and leukocytes
   D. Leukocytes, erythrocytes, and thrombocytes

5. **What is the purpose of an electrocardiogram?**
   A. Indicate the rate of blood flow
   B. Display the heart's rate and rhythm
   C. Identify a person's blood group type
   D. Determine cell type in a blood sample

6. **Which represents the correct order of airflow in the lungs?**
   A. Bronchi, trachea, alveoli, bronchioles
   B. Alveoli, bronchioles, bronchi, trachea
   C. Trachea, bronchi, bronchioles, alveoli
   D. Bronchioles, alveoli, trachea, bronchi

7. **What process does the respiratory system use to facilitate gas exchange in and out of the lungs?**
   A. Diffusion
   B. Exhalation
   C. Inspiration
   D. Ventilation

8. **What is the function of the pharynx?**
   A. Allow food and air to pass into the body
   B. Warm and moisten air during inhalation
   C. Create a chest cavity at the base of the lungs
   D. Provide structural support to the alveolar region

9. **After a person eats birthday cake, which of the following enzymes is needed to break down the sucrose in the cake?**
   A. Lactase
   B. Maltase
   C. Peptidase
   D. Sucrase

10. What is the benefit of the stomach lining being covered with rugae?

   A. Rugae increase the output of gastric juices.

   B. Rugae increase the surface area of the stomach.

   C. Rugae increase the permeability of the stomach walls.

   D. Rugae increase the types of nutrients that can diffuse.

11. What organ of the body compensates when a person's intake of vitamins decreases?

   A. Appendix   C. Pancreas

   B. Liver   D. Stomach

12. Where is the cervix located?

   A. top of the uterus

   B. top of the ovaries

   C. bottom of the vagina

   D. bottom of the uterus

13. The first trimester of gestation corresponds roughly to which developmental process?

   A. Embryogenesis

   B. Fertilization

   C. Meiosis

   D. Menstruation

14. How does the developing fetus primarily eliminate metabolic wastes?

   A. A developing fetus does not produce metabolic wastes.

   B. Fetal waste is excreted as feces, which pass into the mother's anus.

   C. Fetal waste is passed down the umbilical cord to the mother's circulatory system.

   D. Fetal waste is passed down the umbilical cord and leaves the mother's body via the vagina.

15. Which of the following correctly orders the route of a fetus during childbirth?

   A. Uterus cervix vagina

   B. Cervix uterus vagina

   C. Uterus vas deferens vagina

   D. Ovary Fallopian tube uterus

16. Which of the following symptoms related to kidney function is displayed with an impaired posterior pituitary gland?

   A. Thirst   C. Weight gain

   B. Tiredness   D. Concentrated urine

17. When is urine formed?

   A. after fluid reaches the bladder.

   B. when fluid fills the collecting duct.

   C. before blood enters the glomerulus.

   D. during fluid transport to the urethra.

18. At which of the following ages would ossification most likely take place to replace cartilage at the growth plate?

   A. 5   C. 42

   B. 18   D. 91

19. Which structure protects the lungs?

    A. femur
    B. ribcage
    C. scapula
    D. skull

20. Which muscle causes a joint to bend?

    A. Cardiac
    B. Extension
    C. Flexor
    D. Smooth

21. What substance is required to drive the slide filament process?

    A. ATP
    B. Hormone
    C. Potassium
    D. Water

22. The hair _____ is not attached to the follicle.

    A. bulb
    B. root
    C. shaft
    D. strand

23. Which type of tissue is the hypodermis primarily composed of?

    A. adipose
    B. connective
    C. epithelial
    D. muscle

24. What type of cells are actively growing within the hair bulb?

    A. basal
    B. epidermal
    C. epithelial
    D. merkel

25. What is a major structure of the limbic system?

    A. Brainstem
    B. Spinal cord
    C. Hypothalamus
    D. Cerebral cortex

26. Which of the following is a characteristic of an interneuron?

    A. Forms neural circuits
    B. Interacts with effectors
    C. Sends impulses to the CNS
    D. Functions as an efferent nerve cell

27. What structure is directly involved in gas exchange?

    A. Alveolus
    B. Bronchiole
    C. Pharynx
    D. Trachea

28. Some intercellular chemical signals diffuse across cell membranes and bind to intracellular receptors. What are the two factors that enable this to occur?

    A. They are small and soluble.
    B. They are large and soluble.
    C. They are small and insoluble.
    D. They are large and insoluble.

29. Which of the following hormones would cause skin color to become darker?

    A. Follicle-stimulating
    B. Growth-stimulating
    C. Thyroid-stimulating
    D. Melanocyte-stimulating

30. Not all cells in the pancreas secrete insulin because of the hormone somatostatin, which inhibits the release of insulin by all cells. What type of intercellular chemical signal does this illustrate?

    A. Autocrine
    B. Neuromodulator
    C. Paracrine
    D. Pheromone

31. Why is it necessary to have an extensive network of blood vessels supplied in the endocrine glands?

    A. Because glands filter waste from the blood

    B. Because the glands empty directly into the blood

    C. Because blood empties into the endocrine system

    D. Because blood filters waste from the endocrine glands

32. A laboratory technician identifies a person's blood as O+. What does this mean?

    A. The person can accept type AB blood.

    B. Antibodies are found in the blood's plasma.

    C. An Rh factor is on the red blood cells' surface.

    D. Antibodies bind to antigens in the blood sample.

33. What is the smallest contractile unit of skeletal muscle?

    A. Actin

    B. Epimysium

    C. Myofibril

    D. Sarcomere

34. Why is vascular spasm important?

    A. Initiates blood coagulation

    B. Restricts platelet aggregation

    C. Reduces blood flow to an injured site

    D. Signals for the body to end wound healing

35. What is a benefit of a taxonomic system?

    A. Researchers can describe how living things behave.

    B. Researchers can develop names for new organisms.

    C. Living things can be distinguished from nonliving things.

    D. Living things can be classified based on their molecular traits.

36. A study was performed to evaluate which type of road salt deiced a road most quickly. What is the independent variable?

    A. Deicing time period

    B. Road used for deicing

    C. Type of road salt used

    D. Amount of road salt used

37. Which statement confirms that the cell membrane is selectively permeable?

    A. Receptors are found on a cell's surface.

    B. Cells communicate with each other using cell signals.

    C. Environmental changes can cause a cell to expand or shrink.

    D. Sodium ions must travel through ion channels to enter the cell.

38. Which structure do cells rely on for movement?

    A. Flagellum   C. Pili

    B. Microtubule   D. Vesicle

39. Which of the following is most likely absent in prokaryotic cells?

    A. Cilia   C. Lysosomes

    B. Flagella   D. Ribosomes

40. If a biochemist isolates a large amount of pyruvate, which part of the cell is he working with?

   A. Chloroplasts   C. Mitochondria

   B. Cytoplasm   D. Nucleus

41. Which gives the correct order of cellular respiration?

   A. Glycolysis, Acetyl-CoA, Citric Acid Cycle, Electron Transport Chain

   B. Citric Acid Cycle, Glycolysis, Acetyl-CoA, Electron Transport Chain

   C. Glycolysis, Acetyl-CoA, Electron Transport Chain, Citric Acid Cycle

   D. Glycolysis, Citric Acid Cycle, Electron Transport Chain, Acetyl-CoA

42. During which phase of meiosis do chiasmata structures form?

   A. Prophase I   C. Metaphase I

   B. Prophase II   D. Metaphase II

43. A _____ is a rod-shaped structure that forms when a single DNA molecule and its associated proteins coil tightly before cell division.

   A. centromere   C. chromosome

   B. chromatid   D. gene

44. Which of the following is the base that will bind with cytosine?

   A. Adenine   C. Guanine

   B. Cytosine   D. Thymine

45. Which term is used interchangeably with *negative variation*?

   A. Non-correlation

   B. Direct correlation

   C. Inverse correlation

   D. Positive correlation

46. A fish in a large fish tank is fed 5 ounces of food once a day. The same type of fish in a second tank is fed 10 ounces of food each day. The same type of fish in a third tank is fed 2 ounces of food four times a day. This study lasts for a four-week period where fish weight is measured weekly. What is the dependent variable?

   A. Weight of the fish

   B. Type of food used

   C. Number of fish tanks

   D. Frequency of feedings

47. Five tropical plants are kept at varying humidity levels in a greenhouse for three months. One plant is left outside in normal conditions. Plant height is measured weekly. What is the control of the experiment?

   A. Plant height for each tropical plant

   B. The plant left outside in normal conditions

   C. Humidity level readings in the greenhouse

   D. Amount of time used to study plant height

48. A neutral atom of which element has 2 electrons in the first shell and 6 electrons in the second shell of the electron cloud?

   A. Beryllium   C. Helium

   B. Carbon   D. Oxygen

49. An atom has 17 protons, 20 neutrons, and 17 electrons. What is its mass, in amu?

   A. 17   C. 37

   B. 20   D. 54

50. A neutral atom of aluminum has 13 electrons. How many electrons can be found in each shell in the electron cloud?

   A. 6 in the first shell, 7 in the second shell

   B. 2 in the first shell, 11 in the second shell

   C. 2 in the first shell, 8 in the second shell, 3 in the third shell

   D. 3 in the first shell, 5 in the second shell, 5 in the third shell

51. As a substance _____, the particles in the substance get closer together.

   A. boils   C. melts

   B. condenses   D. sublimes

52. What would happen if an amino acid could not pass through a lipid bilayer?

   A. The solutes would be targeted by nearby ions.

   B. The solutes on one side would form a channel to move through.

   C. The amino acid solutes would bond with water and move through the bilayer.

   D. The polar solute particles would form hydrogen bonds with the water molecules surrounding them.

53. _____ is the diffusion of water molecules through a membrane in the direction of higher solute concentration.

   A. Melting   C. Polarity

   B. Osmosis   D. Sublimation

SECTION IV. ENGLISH AND LANGUAGE USAGE

You have 28 minutes to complete 28 questions.

1. **What is the correct plural of** *century*?

   A. Centurys   C. Centuries

   B. Centures   D. Centuryies

2. **Which word(s) in the following sentence should be capitalized?**

   she asked, "do you like indian food?"

   A. she and do

   B. do and indian

   C. she and indian

   D. she, do, and indian

3. **What is missing from the following sentence?**

   He asked, When is the assignment due?

   A. There should be quotation marks.

   B. There needs to be a semicolon after *asked*.

   C. There should be a comma after *assignment*.

   D. Nothing is missing.

4. **Which is the correct plural form of the noun** *class*?

   A. Class   C. Class's

   B. Class'   D. Classes

5. **Which pronoun would <u>not</u> work in the following sentence?**

   I asked ____ colleague to bring it to you.

   A. my   C. your

   B. our   D. whose

6. **Which of the following nouns is described by the adjectives "strong" and "healthy" in this sentence?**

   Two weeks after his surgery, Henry felt <u>strong</u> and <u>healthy</u>.

   A. weeks   C. surgery

   B. his   D. Henry

7. **Which of the following book titles does NOT contain a preposition?**

   A. *The Man in the Brown Suit*

   B. *The Secret of Chimneys*

   C. *Murder on the Orient Express*

   D. *And Then There Were None*

8. **What verb tense are the underlined words in the following sentence?**

   The doctor prescribed medicine after my son <u>had been</u> sick for four days.

   A. Past perfect

   B. Present perfect

   C. Past progressive

   D. Present progressive

9. **Which of the following subjects correctly agrees with the verb "has" in this sentence?**

   Everyone I know <u>has</u> the day off, but my boss wants me to work.

   A. Everyone   C. day

   B. I   D. boss

10. **Which of the following verbs correctly completes this sentence?**

    The girls on the team ____ excited to play in the championships.

    A. is

    B. am

    C. are

    D. ares

11. **Which of the following uses a conjunction to combine the sentences below so the focus is on puppies requiring a lot of work?**

    Puppies are fun-loving animals. They do require a lot of work.

    A. Puppies are fun-loving animals; they do require a lot of work.

    B. Puppies are fun-loving animals, so they do require a lot of work.

    C. Since puppies are fun-loving animals they do require a lot of work.

    D. Although puppies are fun-loving animals, they do require a lot of work.

12. **Which of the following is an example of a complex sentence?**

    A. Tabitha tried rock climbing, having a fear of heights.

    B. Tabitha tried rock climbing; having a fear of heights.

    C. Tabitha tried rock climbing and having a fear of heights.

    D. Tabitha tried rock climbing despite having a fear of heights.

13. **How would you connect the following clauses?**

    He ate a lot on vacation.

    He did not gain any weight.

    A. He ate a lot on vacation if he did not gain any weight.

    B. He ate a lot on vacation, but he did not gain any weight.

    C. He ate a lot on vacation since he did not gain any weight.

    D. He ate a lot on vacation because he did not gain any weight.

14. **Identify the type of clause.**

    I ate, and he drank.

    A. Coordinate clause

    B. Dependent clause

    C. Subordinate clause

    D. Independent clause

15. **Fill in the blank with the correct subordinating conjunction.**

    _____ the class was difficult, Allison passed with flying colors.

    A. If

    B. Since

    C. Because

    D. Although

16. **Which of the following sentences uses the MOST formal language?**

    A. I can't come to your party.

    B. I will be unable to come to your party.

    C. I won't be able to go to your party.

    D. I can't go to your party.

17. **In which of the following situations would it be best to use informal language?**

    A. In a seminar

    B. Writing a postcard

    C. Talking to your boss

    D. Participating in a professional conference

18. In which of the following situations would you use formal language?

    A. Texting a friend

    B. A family reunion

    C. Skyping your grandparents

    D. At a Parent-Teacher meeting

19. Which of the following root words means far?

    A. tele

    B. trans

    C. post

    D. ante

20. What is the best definition of the word translucent?

    A. Blocking all light

    B. Blinding with light

    C. Giving off colorful light

    D. Letting some light through

21. Monochromatic most nearly means

    A. having one color

    B. having many parts

    C. having a lot of time

    D. having too much heat

22. What is the best definition of the word veritable?

    A. Noble

    B. Genuine

    C. Forceful

    D. Exaggerated

23. Which of the following prefixes means with?

    A. bio-

    B. per-

    C. con-

    D. trans-

24. Which of the following words in this sentence has more than one meaning?

    Javier was overjoyed when he finally finished his application for college.

    A. Overjoyed

    B. Finally

    C. Application

    D. College

25. Which of the following is the meaning of "bass" as used in this sentence?

    Natalie's fingers were calloused after practicing her bass.

    A. Kind of fish

    B. Low and deep sound

    C. Lowest male singing voice

    D. A guitar with four strings that makes low sounds

26. Which of the following context clues correctly helps you define the word "formula" in this sentence?

    The mother gave her baby his formula after he woke up from his nap in the car.

    A. "mother"

    B. "baby"

    C. "nap"

    D. "car"

27. Which of the following is the meaning of "somnambulist" as used in this sentence?

    If you wake up outside in your pajamas in the middle of the night, you may be a somnambulist.

    A. Explorer

    B. Magician

    C. Insomniac

    D. Sleepwalker

28. **Which of the following context clues correctly helps you define the word "pungent" in this sentence?**

The <u>pungent</u> odor in the room made everyone's eyes tear for a few minutes.

A. "odor"   C. "made"

B. "room"   D. "tear"

TEAS Practice Exam 6
Answer Key with Explanatory Answers

Section I. Reading

1. B. The main idea of the sentence is how kindergarten has changed. **Skill: Main Ideas, Topic Sentences, and Supporting Details.**

2. A. The sentence conveys information about today's kindergartens being more like first grade classrooms from thirty years ago. This makes it most likely to fit into a persuasive paragraph about kindergarten not being developmentally appropriate for children. **Skill: Main Ideas, Topic Sentences, and Supporting Details.**

3. C. If the sentence were a topic sentence, its supporting details would likely share information to develop the idea that kindergarten today looks very different from kindergarten years ago. **Skill: Main Ideas, Topic Sentences, and Supporting Details.**

4. D. A summary is a restatement of the main ideas of a text. Summaries also use different words to restate these main ideas. **Skill: Summarizing Text and Using Text Features.**

5. A. A diagram presents a picture with labels that show the parts of an object or functions of a mechanism. This would be the best graphic to support the paragraph mentioned. **Skill: Summarizing Text and Using Text Features.**

6. D. A pie chart is useful for representing all of something – in this case a large donation made to a charity – and the percentage values of its parts. **Skill: Summarizing Text and Using Text Features.**

7. A. The main point is the unifying idea. Here, that is the argument that there is a need for diverse superheroes. **Skill: The Writing Process.**

8. C. The author of this outline has not yet figured out how to grab the attention and set up the topic in the introductory paragraph. The introduction in this outline contains only the thesis statement. **Skill: The Writing Process.**

9. A. The sentence about the world needing more heroes is a surprising statement that could grab the reader's attention at the beginning of the essay. **Skill: The Writing Process.**

10. C. A new body paragraph needs to say something new, not just restate the points already made. However, it must also stay focused on the main point about superheroes, not veer off onto a related side topic. **Skill: The Writing Process.**

11. C. This outline contains information from research, and the writer has made a note of where the quotations came from. This will help later when it is time to create citations. **Skill: The Writing Process.**

2. **A.** Prewriting takes place before the writing. Revising is the process of making major changes to the content and structure of a draft after it is written. **Skill: The Writing Process.**

3. **C.** Objects uncovered at an archeological dig are artifacts. They are also things, but *thing* is even less precise than *object*. **Skill: Essay Revision and Transitions.**

4. **A.** Choosing more precise language often makes writing stronger. However, you should be aware of your audience's likely needs. Small children might not know the word *artifact*, so it's best to go with a simpler choice (unless you're actively teaching archeological terms). **Skill: Essay Revision and Transitions.**

5. **C.** Coherent writing is logical and consistent, so that readers can follow the flow of ideas. **Skill: Essay Revision and Transitions.**

6. **B.** The phrase *until recently* and the word *now* connect ideas in these sentences by showing when people believed the ideas expressed. **Skill: Essay Revision and Transitions.**

7. **C.** Wordy phrases should generally be avoided if it is possible to convey the same idea with fewer words. The phrase "due to the fact that" means *because,* and the phrase "on the other hand" means *however.* **Skill: Essay Revision and Transitions.**

8. **B.** The author of this passage is reporting on a controversial issue with an objective or impartial tone. **Skill: Tone, Mood, and Transition Words.**

9. **C.** Dr. Hussein's words show that he cares deeply about the responsibility of his position. His tone could be described as earnest or concerned. **Skill: Tone, Mood, and Transition Words.**

20. **A.** Liz Goode is highly critical of embryonic research. Her tone could be described as harsh, scathing, or critical. **Skill: Tone, Mood, and Transition Words.**

21. **D.** The phrase "on the contrary" helps express a contrast. In other words, it introduces a juxtaposition of dissimilar ideas. **Skill: Tone, Mood, and Transition Words.**

22. **B.** Phrases like "for instance" help introduce examples in writing. **Skill: Tone, Mood, and Transition Words.**

23. **C.** A transition is a word or phrase that links ideas. The word "also" is a transition meant to introduce an additional idea on a topic. **Skill: Tone, Mood, and Transition Words.**

24. **D.** The sentences would be best served with an example transition and an addition transition. **Skill: Tone, Mood, and Transition Words.**

25. **A.** Transition words like "despite" express a contrast between ideas. **Skill: Tone, Mood, and Transition Words.**

26. **C.** If the article argues a point, it is meant to persuade. **Skill: Understanding Author's Purpose, Point of View, and Rhetorical Strategies.**

27. D. Entertaining texts tell stories. This story is about one family's experience moving to a foreign country. **Skill: Understanding Author's Purpose, Point of View, and Rhetorical Strategies.**

28. C. This is a book review. Although it includes some information about the story, its primary purpose is to convince you to read it. This makes it a persuasive text. **Skill: Understanding Author's Purpose, Point of View, and Rhetorical Strategies.**

29. C. Most of the information despite the second paragraph is not verifiable, but the fact that the book chronicles the final years of Audrey Lacoste's life is a fact. **Skill: Understanding Author's Purpose, Point of View, and Rhetorical Strategies.**

30. C. This is a book review. The author includes details about Audrey Lacoste's life to personalize the idea of getting old by telling one individual's struggle. This is meant to appeal to the reader's emotions. **Skill: Understanding Author's Purpose, Point of View, and Rhetorica Strategies.**

31. C. The Rim Trail is the dotted line running generally north-south past the Lodge in the middle. Fairyland Point is in the far north, so a walk north on the trail would get you there. **Skill: Evaluating and Integrating Data.**

32. D. Inspiration Point is between Sunset Point and Bryce Point along the Rim Trail. **Skill: Evaluating and Integrating Data.**

33. A. The main road parallels the Rim Trail but only touches the northernmost and southernmost viewpoints; it does not touch Sunset Point. **Skill: Evaluating and Integrating Data.**

34. D. The compass shows that the left-hand side of the page is west. The Visitor's Center is the westernmost labeled point on the map. **Skill: Evaluating and Integrating Data.**

35. A. The legend explains what the solid and dotted lines represent. In this case, the dotted line is a trail and the solid line is a road. **Skill: Evaluating and Integrating Data.**

36. A. If Carla wants to limit her calorie intake, she needs to know not only how many calories are in a serving of the foods and drinks she consumes, but also the number of servings per package or bottle. **Skill: Evaluating and Integrating Data.**

37. A. The index tells which subtopics are covered on which pages of a book. **Skill: Evaluating and Integrating Data.**

38. A. This first statement is an opinion since it reflects someone's beliefs about doctors. **Skill: Facts, Opinions, and Evaluating an Argument.**

39. B. This passage argues that teens and young adults spend too much time on social media. **Skill: Facts, Opinions, and Evaluating an Argument.**

40. B. Factual information is verifiable and not based on personal beliefs or feelings. The statistic about the number of teens who go online daily is a fact. **Skill: Facts, Opinions, and Evaluating an Argument.**

41. A. This statement takes a complex issue and presents it as if only two possible options are in play. This is an either/or fallacy. **Skill: Facts, Opinions, and Evaluating an Argument.**

42. B. This sentence makes an overgeneralization by claiming that online interactions are never as good as conversations with human beings. It is possible to imagine many exceptions to this statement. **Skill: Facts, Opinions, and Evaluating an Argument.**

43. C. The sentence in question is an example of circular reasoning. That is, it restates the argument in different words instead of providing evidence to back it up. **Skill: Facts, Opinions, and Evaluating an Argument.**

44. A. The phrase "too much" in this sentence reflects a judgment that is subject to interpretation. This indicates that the sentence reflects a belief rather than a fact. **Skill: Facts, Opinions, and Evaluating an Argument.**

45. A. Adelia is attempting to call a pet, not a child. You can infer this because she calls Mr. Snuggles "vermin" and bangs on a bowl with a spoon to get his attention. **Skill: Understanding Primary Sources, Making Inferences, and Drawing Conclusions.**

46. B. Adelia's bathrobe is not evidence that she is frustrated at Mr. Snuggles. **Skill: Understanding Primary Sources, Making Inferences, and Drawing Conclusions.**

47. A. Adelia tries repeatedly to call Mr. Snuggles, and when he does not come, she goes out to look for him. This implies that she does care about him, even if she is angry at him. **Skill: Understanding Primary Sources, Making Inferences, and Drawing Conclusions.**

48. C. The line about Raul and his plants does not explicitly say Adelia is babysitting Mr. Snuggles, but it suggests that she is caring for the pet for someone else. **Skill: Understanding Primary Sources, Making Inferences, and Drawing Conclusions.**

49. B. A biography of Anne Frank would be a historical or analytical account that added insight on the topic. This makes it a secondary source. **Skill: Understanding Primary Sources, Making Inferences, and Drawing Conclusions.**

50. D. Primary sources are written by people who witnessed the original creation or discovery of the information they present. This description does not apply to an encyclopedia entry. **Skill: Understanding Primary Sources, Making Inferences, and Drawing Conclusions.**

51. C. This passage is an explanation of phone habits in two eras. Although it uses a few time words, it does not describe narrative scenes. It is an expository piece. **Skill: Types of Passages, Text Structures, Genre and Theme.**

52. D. The passage describes phone use in two eras, highlighting similarities and differences. This makes it a compare/contrast piece. **Skill: Types of Passages, Text Structures, Genre and Theme.**

53. A. This piece describes parts of both the author's life and another person's life, but it is not an autobiography or biography because it is not telling a story of either one. Rather, it is an essay—short description of a subject from the author's point of view. **Skill: Types of Passages, Text Structures, Genre and Theme.**

Section II. Mathematics

1. C. The correct solution is that 60 percent of the students like pandas and monkeys: 33.33% plus 26.67% equals 60%. **Skill: Interpreting Graphics.**

2. C. The correct solution is $2\frac{1}{2}$ because $2\frac{2}{3}-\frac{1}{6}=\frac{8}{3}-\frac{1}{6}=\frac{16}{6}-\frac{1}{6}=\frac{15}{6}=2\frac{3}{6}=2\frac{1}{2}$. **Skill: Addition and Subtraction of Fractions.**

3. B. The value of the home is $350,000 because $\frac{100}{18}=\frac{X}{\$63,000}$ and x = $350,000. **Skill: Ratios, Proportions, and Percentages.**

4. D. The interest rate is 42.4% because $\frac{\$212}{\$500}=\frac{X}{100}$ and X = 0.424, which means the annual interest rate was 42.4%. **Skill: Ratios, Proportions, and Percentages.**

5. A. The ratio is 4:11. A ratio is like a fraction of two numbers, although in this case the answer uses colon notation. The ratio of brand B to brand A is the number of brand-B cars divided by the number of brand-A cars. Reduce to lowest terms: $\frac{48}{132}=\frac{4}{11}$. **Skill: Ratios, Proportions, and Percentages.**

6. D. The correct solution is two bins have the same frequency. The bins 400–600 and 800–1,000 have three friends. **Skill: Interpreting Categorical and Quantitative Data.**

7. C. The ratio is 23:35. The first part of the ratio is the number of people in group Y, which is 230. The second part is the number of people in either group, which is the sum 120 + 230 = 350. The ratio is therefore 230:350 = 23:35. **Skill: Ratios, Proportions, and Percentages.**

8. B. The correct solution is $4\frac{5}{12}$ because $5\frac{2}{3}-1\frac{1}{4}=5\frac{8}{12}-1\frac{3}{12}=4\frac{5}{12}$ feet. **Skill: Solving Real World Mathematical Problems.**

9. D. The correct answer is D. Although solving each proportion is one approach, the easiest approach is to compare them as they are. The proportions in answers A and B yield the same number for the unknown because they keep the same numbers in either the numerators or the denominators. Answer C just reverses the order of the equation in answer A, which does not yield a different number for the unknown. Answer D flips one fraction without flipping the other, which changes the proportion. **Skill: Ratios, Proportions, and Percentages.**

10. A. The correct solution is the interquartile range is greater for Team 2 by 1 point. The interquartile range is 12 points for Team 1 and 13 points for Team 2. The interquartile range is greater by 1 point for Team 2. **Skill: Interpreting Categorical and Quantitative Data.**

11. C. The correct solution is $(4x + 11)(4x-11)$. The expression $16x^2-121$ is rewritten as $(4x + 11)(4x-11)$ because the value of a is $4x$ and the value of b is 11. **Skill: Polynomials.**

12. C. The correct answer is 7.65 because $\frac{13}{20} = 13.00 \div 20 = 0.65$. **Skill: Decimals and Fractions.**

13. D. The rate of change is 126 inches per month. One approach is to set up a proportion.

$$\frac{1\ day}{4.2\ inches} = \frac{30\ days}{?}$$

Since 1 month is equivalent to 30 days, multiply the rate of change per day by 30 to get the rate of change per month. 4.2 inches multiplied by 30 is 126 inches. Thus, the growth rate is 126 inches per month. **Skill: Ratios, Proportions, and Percentages.**

14. D. The correct answer is $2\frac{9}{10}$ because 290% as a fraction is $2\frac{90}{100} = 2\frac{9}{10}$. **Skill: Decimals and Fractions**

15. A. The correct solution is 0.147 kiloliters. $147\ L \times \frac{1\ kL}{1,000\ L} = \frac{147}{1,000} = 0.147\ kL$. **Skill: Standards of Measure.**

16. A. The student athlete has to travel 15 miles in 20 minutes to give him enough time to change before work. He will need to go (15 miles ÷ 20 minutes) x 60 minutes in an hour = 45 mph. **Skill: Solving Real World Mathematical Problems.**

17. C. The correct solution is 6.

$\frac{x}{2} = 3$ Subtract 5 from both sides of the equation.

$x = 6$ Multiply both sides of the equation by 2.

Skill: Equations with One Variable.

18. B. The correct solution is $1\frac{1}{5}$ because $\frac{2}{5} \times \frac{3}{1} = \frac{6}{5} = 1\frac{1}{5}$. **Skill: Multiplication and Division of Fractions.**

19. C. The correct solution is C because the bar graph displays the values of the revenue and expenses correctly. **Skill: Interpreting Graphics.**

20. C. The man needs 20 feet of wood, which converts into 240 inches while the wood is sold in 18- inch pieces. He'll need 14 pieces of wood to border his garden. **Skill: Multiplication and Division of Fractions.**

21. B. The taxi fare will cost $107.70 because $6.00 + ($5.65 x 18 miles) = $107.70. The equation that properly represents this cost is $5.65m + $6.00= $107.70. **Skill: Solving Real World Mathematical Problems.**

22. C. The correct solution is $9\frac{3}{5}$ because $2\frac{2}{5} \times 4 = \frac{12}{5} \times \frac{4}{1} = \frac{48}{5} = 9\frac{3}{5}$ pounds of apples. **Skill: Solving Real World Mathematical Problems.**

23. B. The correct solution is 8 because $x^3 = 27 + 5 = 32 \div 4 = 8$. **Skill: Equations with One Variable.**

24. D. The nurse's overtime rate is $23.94 an hour because $21 x 1.14 = $23.94. Her normal salary is $840 because $21 x 40 = $840, so her paycheck is $840 + ($23.94 x 12) = $1,127.28. **Skill: Decimals and Fractions.**

25. B. The correct answer is $\frac{1}{14}$ because $\frac{3}{14} \times \frac{1}{3} = \frac{3}{42} = \frac{1}{14}$. **Skill: Multiplication and Division of Fractions.**

26. A. The manager would have to pay $43.75 because $\frac{1}{6} = \frac{X}{\$262.52}$ and x = $43.75. **Skill: Ratios, Proportions, and Percentages.**

27. D. The correct solution is 200.96. The radius is 8 centimeters and $A = \pi r^2 \approx 3.14(8)^2 \approx 3.14(64) \approx 200.96$ square centimeters. **Skill: Circles.**

28. C. The correct solution is $\frac{2}{3}$.

$3x + 2 + 9 = 6x + 9$	Multiply all terms by the least common denominator of 3 to eliminate the fractions.
$3x + 11 = 6x + 9$	Combine like terms on the left side of the equation.
$-3x + 11 = 9$	Subtract $6x$ from both sides of the equation.
$-3x = -2$	Subtract 11 from both sides of the equation.
$x = \frac{2}{3}$	Divide both sides of the equation by -3.

Skill: Equations with One Variable.

29. C. The team must run 5 laps because $4 \div \frac{8}{10} = \frac{4}{1} \times \frac{10}{8} = \frac{40}{8} = 5$. **Skill: Multiplication and Division of Fractions.**

30. C. Justin is spending $\frac{1}{3}$ of his week working because he spends 56 hours at work out of 168 hours of the week. The fraction $\frac{56}{168}$ can be reduced to $\frac{1}{3}$. **Skill: Decimals and Fractions.**

31. D. The correct solution is entertainment and homework total is the same as the amount of time in school because the sum of entertainment and homework is 25%. **Skill: Interpreting Graphics.**

32. A. The correct solution is 3 because the equation simplifies to 5x = 15 and x = 3. **Skill: Equations with One Variable.**

33. A. The correct solution is 7.8125 gallons. $1{,}000 \text{ fl oz} \times \frac{1 \text{ pt}}{16 \text{ fl oz}} \times \frac{1 \text{ qt}}{2 \text{ pt}} \times \frac{1 \text{ gal}}{4 \text{ qt}} = \frac{1{,}000}{128} = 7.8125 \text{ gal}$. **Skill: Standards of Measure.**

34. B. Using the appropriate conversion formula, $12°C \times \frac{9}{5} = 21.6 + 32 = 53.6°F$ which is rounded up to 54°F. **Skill: Standards of Measure.**

35. C. The correct solution is $6\frac{1}{12}$ because $2\frac{3}{4} + 3\frac{1}{3} = 2\frac{9}{12} + 3\frac{4}{12} = 5\frac{13}{12} = 6\frac{1}{12}$ miles. **Skill: Solving Real World Mathematical Problems.**

36. A. The girl took $\frac{1}{7}$ of the box because $\frac{8}{56} = \frac{1}{7}$. **Skill: Decimals and Fractions.**

Section III. Science

1. B. This is a negative feedback mechanism because its goal is to readjust the internal environment to return it to a steady, constant, healthy state. **Skill: Organization of the Human Body.**

2. A. The dorsal cavity has two subdivisions: the cranial cavity and the spinal cavity. **Skill: Organization of the Human Body.**

3. D. In a supine position, a person is lying flat with the face and torso facing upward. **Skill: Organization of the Human Body.**

4. C. Thrombocytes, erythrocytes, and leukocytes are formed elements found in blood. Erythrocytes are the smallest with a cell diameter of 0.008 millimeters, while leukocytes are the largest with a cell diameter of 0.02 millimeters. **Skill: Cardiovascular System.**

5. B. An electrocardiogram records a person's heart rate and rhythm to evaluate how well the heart functions. **Skill: Cardiovascular System.**

6. C. After air reaches the trachea, it travels through the bronchi, which branch into bronchioles before reaching the alveolar region of the lungs. **Skill: The Respiratory System.**

7. D. Pulmonary ventilation is the act of breathing, or respiration. The respiratory system uses this process to bring air into and out of the lungs. **Skill: The Respiratory System.**

8. A. The pharynx is found right behind the nasal cavity. It is a passageway through which food and air flow. Skill: **The Respiratory System.**

9. D. Sucrase is the enzyme that breaks down sucrose. **Skill: Gastrointestinal System.**

10. B. Rugae increase the surface area of the interior of the stomach. **Skill: Gastrointestinal System.**

11. B. One function of the liver is to store vitamins. **Skill: Gastrointestinal System.**

12. D. The cervix joins the bottom of the uterus to the top of the vagina. **Skill: Reproductive System.**

13. A. Embryogenesis takes place over the first 11–12 weeks after fertilization, which corresponds with the first trimester of pregnancy. **Skill: Reproductive System.**

14. C. Fetal waste primarily passes through the umbilical cord into the mother's circulatory system, where it is removed primarily by the mother's kidneys. There is no mechanical

connection between the fetus and the mother's anus or vagina; the fetus produces a large amount of metabolic waste. **Skill: Reproductive System.**

15. A. The fetus completes gestation in the uterus. Then, it passes through the cervix and out of the vagina during childbirth. The ovary and Fallopian tube are not involved in childbirth. The vas deferens is a component of the male reproductive system. **Skill: Reproductive System.**

16. A. Hallmarks of ADH secretion impairment are frequent thirst and diluted urine. Because ADH is not communicating well with the kidneys, the collecting ducts are less permeable to water, which causes more water to be excreted than reabsorbed. This is why people with an impaired posterior pituitary gland also experience frequent urination. **Skill: The Urinary System.**

17. B. Urinary formation begins when blood flows through the renal arteries to the kidneys. Once this blood reaches the glomerulus in nephrons, it is filtered through various tubules before accumulating in the collecting duct. At the collecting duct, once all substances are reabsorbed, the leftover byproduct is urine. **Skill: The Urinary System.**

18. A. Ossification is the process of generating new bone tissue by filling in cartilage with mineral deposits to harden the cartilage. Growth plates are present near the ends of long bones. They are sites where ossification occurs so that a child's long bones can grow and the child can get taller. **Skill: Skeletal System.**

19. B. The sternum and ribcage are part of the axial skeleton. They protect the lungs from external damage. **Skill: Skeletal System.**

20. C. Flexor muscles are one part of a skeletal muscle pair that helps bones in the body move. They do so by causing a joint to bend. **Skill: Muscular System.**

21. A. Molecules of ATP are used to energize and reenergize the protein molecules myosin according to the slide filament theory. The myosin myofilaments use ATP to attach their heads to thin actin filaments, pulling the thin filaments closer to the M-line during skeletal muscle contraction. **Skill: Muscular System.**

22. C. The hair shaft is the portion of hair found on the surface of the body. It is not attached to the hair follicle, which is in the dermis. **Skill: Integumentary System.**

23. A. The hypodermis is the subcutaneous layer beneath the dermis. It consists of fat, or adipose tissue, which serves as a layer of insulation deep inside the skin. This region also functions as an energy reservoir, supplying energy to cells. **Skill: Integumentary System.**

24. A. The hair bulb is found deep beneath the skin's surface under the hair root. Within this region, basal cells are actively dividing by mitosis. **Skill: Integumentary System.**

25. C. The limbic system is part of the forebrain, or cerebrum. It consists of four major structures: hypothalamus, hippocampus, amygdala, and thalamus. **Skill: The Nervous System.**

26. A. The interneuron is a type of nerve cell that bridges a connection between motor and sensory neurons to create neural circuits. This bridge facilitates communication between the neurons. **Skill: The Nervous System.**

27. A. The alveolus is a tiny air sac found in the lung. Its primary function is to help the respiratory system perform gas exchange. **Skill: The Respiratory System.**

28. A. To pass through the cell membrane, the chemical signals must be small and soluble. **Skill: Endocrine System.**

29. D. Melanocyte-stimulating hormones increase melanin production to make skin darker. **Skill: Endocrine System.**

30. C. Paracrine chemical signals are released by cells and have effects on other cell types. Somatostatin, secreted by the pancreas, inhibits the release of insulin by other cells in the pancreas. **Skill: Endocrine System.**

31. B. Because the endocrine glands are ductless, they empty hormones directly into the blood. **Skill: Endocrine System.**

32. C. An Rh factor is a protein or antigen found on the surface of red blood cells. A positive sign indicates it is found on the cells' surface. **Skill: Cardiovascular System.**

33. D. Several contractile units called myofibrils are found within a single muscle fiber. Smaller contractile units called sarcomeres make up a myofibril. **Skill: Muscular System**

34. C. Vascular spasm aids in vasoconstriction of the blood vessel to reduce blood flow to the injured site. **Skill: Cardiovascular System.**

35. B. The purpose of a taxonomic system is to classify, describe, and name living things in an organized manner. **Skill: An Introduction to Biology.**

36. C. The type of road salt used is the independent variable because it is the variable that is purposely changed during the study. It is the causative factor in the experiment. **Skill: An Introduction to Biology.**

37. D. Because a cell membrane is selectively permeable, only certain molecules are allowed to enter. For molecules such as sodium ions to enter, they have to travel through specialized channels. **Skill: Cell Structure, Function, and Type.**

38. A. Flagella are tails attached to a cell that aid in locomotion, or movement throughout a cell's external environment. **Skill: Cell Structure, Function, and Type.**

39. C. Higher order or certain organelles are not found in prokaryotic cells. While these cells contain a cytoplasm surrounded by a plasma membrane, flagella for locomotion, and may have ribosomes, all other organelles are absent. This includes lysosomes, which contain digestive enzymes that break down food in eukaryotes. **Skill: Cell Structure, Function, and Type.**

40. B. Pyruvate is produced during the process of glycolysis. Because glycolysis happens in the cytoplasm of the cell, the chemist is most likely working with this structure. **Skill: Cellular Reproduction, Cellular Respiration, and Photosynthesis.**

41. A. A cell produces energy through metabolism by breaking glucose molecules into pyruvate This happens via glycolysis. The pyruvate molecule is prepped for the citric acid cycle by being oxidized to Acetyl-CoA. Once the citric acid cycle happens, the largest amount of energy is generated via the electron transport chain. **Skill: Cellular Reproduction, Cellular Respiration, and Photosynthesis.**

42. A. Chiasmata are X-shaped structures that form when chromosomes from the mother and father of an organism undergoing meiosis are physically bound. This happens during prophase I of meiosis. **Skill: Cellular Reproduction, Cellular Respiration, and Photosynthesis.**

43. C. A chromosome is a rod-shaped structure that forms when a single DNA molecule and its associated proteins coil tightly before cell division. **Skill: Genetics and DNA.**

44. C. Cytosine will only bind with guanine, and vice versa. **Skill: Genetics and DNA.**

45. C. Other terms for *negative variation* are indirect correlation, inverse correlation, and negative correlation. **Skill: Designing an Experiment.**

46. A. The weight of fish is the dependent variable because it is dependent on how much food is supplied to each fish tank over the four-week period. **Skill: Designing an Experiment.**

47. B. The plant left outside is the control because it is not influenced by the independent variable, which is not experimentally manipulated. **Skill: Designing an Experiment.**

48. D. The atom described has a total of 8 electrons. Because it is neutral, it has the same number of protons as electrons. Any atom with 8 protons is oxygen, given by the atomic number in the periodic table. **Skill: Scientific Notation.**

49. C. The mass is determined by adding the numbers of protons and neutrons (17 + 20 = 37). **Skill: Scientific Notation.**

50. C. The electrons are found in the lowest possible shells. Only 2 can fit in the first shell, and only 8 can fit in the second shell. Filling those levels accommodates 10 electrons. The remaining 3 electrons will go into the third shell. **Skill: Scientific Notation.**

51. B. As particles condense, the substance turns from gas to liquid. The particles of liquids are closer together than the particles of gas. **Skill: States of Matter.**

52. D. Unable to cross the membrane, the polar solute particles would form hydrogen bonds with the water molecules surrounding them. **Skill: Properties of Matter.**

53. B. Osmosis is the diffusion of water molecules through a membrane in the direction of higher solute concentration. **Skill: Properties of Matter.**

Section IV. English and Language Usage

1. C. With a word ending in *-y*, you drop the *-y* and add *-ies*. **Skill: Spelling.**

2. D. *she, do,* and *indian. She* is at the beginning of the sentence and needs to be capitalized. *Do* is at the beginning of a quoted sentence and also needs to be capitalized. Nationalities such as Indian should always be capitalized. **Skill: Capitalization.**

3. A. *There should be quotation marks.* Direct quotes from someone else should be enclosed in quotation marks. **Skill: Punctuation.**

4. D. *Classes* is the plural form of the noun *class*. **Skill: Nouns.**

5. D. We are looking for a possessive pronoun. *Whose* is a relative pronoun and can only be used to show possession when the sentence is a question. **Skill: Pronouns.**

6. D. These adjectives describe *Henry*. **Skill: Adjectives and Adverbs.**

7. D. *In, of,* and *on* are prepositions in the other titles. **Skill: Conjunctions and Prepositions.**

8. A. *Had been* is past perfect tense. **Skill: Verbs and Verb Tenses.**

9. A. The verb *has* must agree with the subject *everyone*. **Skill: Subject and Verb Agreement.**

10. C. *Girls* is a third person plural subject, so it takes the verb form *are*. **Skill: Subject and Verb Agreement.**

11. D. The subordinate conjunction "although" combines the sentences and puts the focus on puppies requiring a lot of work. **Skill: Types of Sentences.**

12. D. This is a complex sentence because it has a dependent clause, an independent clause, and a subordinating conjunction, *despite*. **Skill: Types of Sentences.**

13. B. He ate a lot on vacation, but he did not gain any weight. These two clauses are of equal grammatical rank and can be connected with a coordinating conjunction. *But* is the conjunction that makes the most sense. **Skill: Types of Clauses.**

14. A. Coordinate clause. A coordinate clause is a sentence or phrase that combines clauses of equal grammatical rank (verbs, nouns, adjectives, phrases, or independent clauses) by using a coordinating conjunction (and, but, for, nor, or, so, yet). **Skill: Types of Clauses.**

15. D. Although. The word *although* signifies the beginning of a dependent clause and is the only conjunction that makes sense in the sentence. **Skill: Types of Clauses.**

16. B. I will be unable to come to your party. The sentence does not use contractions and uses the most polite and formal vocabulary. **Skill: Formal and Informal Language.**

17. B. Writing a postcard. It is an informal mode of communication between close friends and relatives. **Skill: Formal and Informal Language.**

18. D. At a parent-teacher meeting. It is best to use formal language with a child's teacher to show respect. **Skill: Formal and Informal Language.**

19. A. The root *tele* means "far." Skill: **Root Words, Prefixes, and Suffixes.**

20. D. The prefix *trans* means "across," and the root word *luc* means "light," so *translucent* means "letting some light pass through or across." Skill: **Root Words, Prefixes, and Suffixes.**

21. A. The root *chrom* means "color" and the prefix *mono* means "one," so *monochromatic* means "having one color." Skill: **Root Words, Prefixes, and Suffixes.**

22. B. The root word *veri* means "true," so *veritable* means "genuine." Skill: **Root Words, Prefixes, and Suffixes.**

23. C. The prefix that means "with" is *con-*. Skill: **Root Words, Prefixes, and Suffixes.**

24. C. The word "application" has more than one meaning. **Skill: Context Clues and Multiple Meaning Words.**

25. D. The meaning of <u>bass</u> in the context of this sentence is "a guitar with four strings that makes low sounds." **Skill: Context Clues and Multiple Meaning Words.**

26. B. The meaning of <u>formula</u> in this context is "a liquid that is given to babies." The phrase "baby" helps you figure out which meaning of <u>formula</u> is being used. **Skill: Context Clues and Multiple Meaning Words.**

27. D. The meaning of <u>somnambulist</u> in the context of this sentence is "sleepwalker." **Skill: Context Clues and Multiple Meaning Words.**

28. D. The meaning of <u>pungent</u> in this context is "having a strong smell." The word "tear" helps you figure out the meaning of <u>pungent</u>. **Skill: Context Clues and Multiple Meaning Words.**

CPSIA information can be obtained
at www.ICGtesting.com
Printed in the USA
BVHW081825160520
578519BV00003B/2